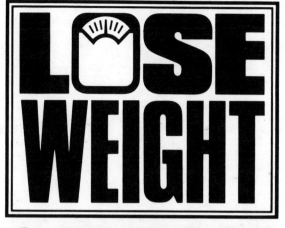

·PREVENTION'S·
LOSE WEIGHT
GUIDEBOOK
·1993·

Edited by Mark Bricklin
and Anne Remondi Imhoff
of *PREVENTION* Magazine

Rodale Press, Emmaus, Pennsylvania

If you have any questions or comments concerning this book, please write:
Rodale Press
Book Readers' Service
33 East Minor Street
Emmaus, PA 18098

ISBN 0-87596-147-9 hardcover
ISSN 1060-9385

Distributed in the book trade by St. Martin's Press

2   4   6   8   10   9   7   5   3   1   hardcover

CONTRIBUTORS

Contributors to *Prevention's Lose Weight Guidebook, 1993*: Covert Bailey; Nick Barton; Frances M. Berg, M.S.; George L. Blackburn, M.D., Ph.D.; Kelly Brownell, Ph.D.; Wayne Callaway, M.D.; Martha Capwell; Michael Castleman; Sonja Connor, M.S., R.N.; William Connor, M.D.; Gail Damerow; Diane Drabinsky, R.D.; Phil Dunphy, P.T.; Stephanie Ebbert; Marise Facher; Howard Flaks, M.D.; Barbara Fritz; Greg Gutfeld; Mary Hubbard, R.D., Ph.D.; Jill J. Jurgensen; Robin Kanarck, Ph.D.; Manfred Kroger, Ph.D.; Michael Lafavore; Ralph LaForge, M.Sc.; Michael R. Lowe, Ph.D.; Susan Luke, M.S., R.D.; Jeff Meade; Melissa Meyers; Mary Carroll Moore; Tom Ney; Cathy Perlmutter; Joseph C. Piscatella; Linda Rao; Marielle Rebuffe-Scrive, Ph.D.; Rodale Food Center staff; Jean Rogers; Maureen Sangiorgio; Joanne Silberner; Marie Simmons; Maria Simonson, Sc.D., Ph.D.; Maggie Spilner; Margo K. Trott; Rena Wing, Ph.D.

Production Editor: Jane Sherman
Book Designer: Linda Brightbill
Copy Editor: Rachel Burd
Executive Editor, *Prevention* Magazine: Emrika Padus
Associate Research Chief, *Prevention* Magazine: Pam Boyer
Office Manager: Roberta Mulliner
Office Personnel: Julie Kehs, Mary Lou Stephen
Photographers of "After" pictures: Jim Osborn (page 189), Gary Pearl (page 196), Thomas Delbeck (page 200), Bill Gillette (page 204)

Packaged by Rapid Transcript, a division of March Tenth, Inc.

NOTICE

The information and ideas in this book are meant to supplement the care and guidance of your physician, not to replace them. The editor cautions you to see a physician before starting any diet or exercise program. An increasing number of physicians are ready to cooperate with patients who want to improve their diet, health and lifestyle. If you are under professional care or are taking medication, we suggest discussing any weight-loss plans with your doctor.

Contents

Good news! This is the year you quit "dieting" *forever* and introduce yourself to permanent weight control. In 1993 we know more than ever about natural weight-loss methods that get results. And there's no better time to take advantage of these breakthrough strategies. *Start here!*

To fight the war on body fat, we need to steer clear of the fat found in food. This year there are more low-fat and no-fat foods on the market than ever before. Eating lean is easier than ever. So here's your personalized step-by-step guide to life in the "light lane."

Check the health of your diet. Choose foods for maximum nutrition, minimum dietary fat, and steady weight loss. With all the variety of foods that you can and should eat for weight loss in the '90s, you finally can *eat* and *be slim!* This chapter shows you how.

Chapter 4: Energize with Exercise: How Fitness Can Boost Fat Loss 103

Here are the fitness activities that will help you achieve the body *you've always wanted.* We'll show you the exercises that burn the most fat and the ones that add great muscle tone. And the best part? With such a wide variety of activities to choose from, it's easier than ever to get started.

Chapter 5: Your Feellngs and Your Physique: The Mind/Body Factor 141

The foolproof formula for losing weight is only complete when you factor in these essential elements: your mind and heart. You can develop *powerful strategies* for beating the stress that leads to overeating. Here are some proven ways to overcome emotional and psychological barriers and achieve *permanent* weight loss.

◆

Chapter 9: The Consumer's Detective Agency: A Revealing Look at the Diet Industry

With all the new diet products on today's market, it's easy to get confused about which ones are safe and reliable. Some are designed to help you take off pounds and others just take you for a ride. So here's a solid-facts evaluation of some of today's popular products and services. It will help you decipher the difference between diet aids and diet gimmicks.

Introducing the MenuMate—a unique chart that will help you design your daily menu. It lists hundreds of foods in order of *how much fat they have in a serving*. For the first time, you can select foods based on how much of your fat budget you're willing to "spend." Plus, you'll have a lot of fun browsing!

Introduction

Every single one of us is a creature of habit: Every day there are many things that we do automatically, without really thinking or trying. And while many of our habits promote our well-being (like looking both ways before we cross a busy street), some of them are clearly bad for us: Maybe we smoke, or bite our nails simply out of the force of habit.

Good and bad habits also extend into the realm of our "dieting" behaviors. Maybe your habit is to eat a doughnut during your morning coffee break or to snack on junk food when you watch TV at night. Or maybe you're not in the habit of exercising. These seem like little things, but linked together, it's these very behaviors that make or break weight-loss success.

In fact, the whole idea behind permanent weight control boils down to one simple principle: You have to change a few habits. Break the bad ones and make more good ones. You could, for example, get in the habit of reading the fat content on the labels before buying foods at the grocery store. Or take up the habit of going to the gym after work. Try breaking the habit of eating when you feel stressed out. Instead, make a habit of going for a brisk 15-minute walk when stress sets in.

Here's a good tip: For every habit you break, take up a new, good habit that's *incompatible* with your bad one. For instance, if you want to break the elevator habit, take up climbing the stairs. Before you know it, your new habit of heading for the stairwell will have completely obliterated your old habit of pushing the elevator button.

With a little repetition and regularity, positive habits are surprisingly easy to nurture. Pretty soon you have a whole system of weight-control practices. Best of all, you'll notice that a few new "little" habits can add up to significant weight loss. And it's completely doable—no gimmicks, no "diets" and no miracles needed. It doesn't even require tremendous willpower.

Where do you start? By changing the way you look at "dieting." You're holding a compilation of the best healthy weight-loss ideas of 1993. We've combed the literature, interviewed the experts and gathered this year's best research discoveries in the science of weight loss. You'll learn new healthwise habits and develop a weight-control *lifestyle* (not a short-term "diet") that will help you uncover the slim, healthy body you have always wanted.

Read through this "best of" collection. Nibble away at it, digesting just a little at a time. Think about what ideas you can most easily set into practice in your life. You'll find that none of the steps toward weight loss is very "hard to swallow." And you'll find that changing your habits can lead to positive changes in your weight, your health, and your self-image—all changes that can improve your whole life! And that can be very habit-forming!

The Editors

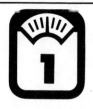

INTRODUCING NATURAL WEIGHT LOSS: DIET NO MORE!

Are You a "Maintainer" or a "Relapser"?

The great American pastime, taking off weight, puts enough strain on most of us who engage in it, but keeping it off—that's the real toughie! We've all seen the TV commercials ("This is me before, and this is me now!"), but what about a couple of years from now? Anyone who loses 20 percent or more of body weight has to work a lot harder at maintaining the lower weight than in taking it off, but a report in the *American Journal of Clinical Nutrition* offers some valuable insights into the problem.

Two groups of women who had lost at least 20 percent of their body weight were studied. Thirty had maintained the loss for at least two years; 44 had reverted to their previous levels. These were some of the factors that made the difference.

Weight-loss strategy. The successful ones were those who had worked out their own programs, reducing their caloric intake without doing away with the foods they enjoyed most, eating more fruits and vegetables and exercising faithfully. The unsuccessful tended to be those who were enrolled in formal weight programs, used diet aids, fasted and avoided favorite foods.

Exercise. Ninety percent of those who maintained their new weight exercised regularly—at least three times weekly and for 30 minutes or more. Fewer than a third of those who regained their weight exercised at all, and with less frequency and effort.

Lifestyle modifications. The successful group were those who understood that maintaining acceptable weight requires a continuing and lifelong change in lifestyle. They monitored their weight, maintained their new eating habits and had no delusions about the effort required to prevent relapse. The others simply assumed that the initial effort was all that was required and were apparently surprised when their weight returned.

Coping strategies. Although the "maintainers" were more apt to deal with stress by meeting it head on and working out rational solutions, the "relapsers" were more likely to use such escape mechanisms as drinking, smoking, eating or sleeping.

Social support. Those who sought help from professional counselors, family or friends had greater success in maintaining their weight loss.

Successful Weight Loss at Any Age

Some things get easier over time. Some things don't—like weight loss. "For a lot of people, when they were 35 or younger, weight was a minor problem," says weight-loss expert and *Prevention* advisor George Blackburn, M.D., Ph.D. "Maybe their clothing was getting a little tighter. But suddenly after age 35, nothing fits. And weight control becomes a struggle for them."

Why do we tend to gain weight with age? There are a lot of powerful reasons. Some are physiological; some are related to lifestyle. But powerful or not, these reasons are not inevitable, unstoppable steamrollers that flatten any weight-control plan after age 35. Weight loss (and weight control) is possible in the middle years—without weird diets and unrealistic fitness schemes that can make your life miserable (and unhealthy).

What's required is a sober look at the 35-plus forces that make weight control so tough, and some equally sober but workable strategies for overcoming them.

Problem Weight Factors

Metabolic Tricks

"One reason that we gain weight with age," says Kelly Brownell, Ph.D., *Prevention* advisor and professor of psychology at Yale University, "is that our metabolism naturally slows over the years—at a rate of 5 percent every ten years, beginning around age 30. This, of course, means fewer calories burned over time, with more calories then stored as fat on the body, if food intake remains constant." The process is compounded because body fat itself burns fewer calories than lean tissue does.

The No-Time-for-Exercise Lifestyle

Weight gain past 35 has a lot to do with the decline in exercise that comes with age. Beginning in their thirties, many people find themselves impossibly busy—yet less physically active than ever before.

Michael Lowe, Ph.D., a clinical psychologist at Hahnemann University in Philadelphia, says, "As we get older we're more likely to get a 'crowded' lifestyle. We're taking care of parents and children and, if we're moving upward in a profession, we have more job demands—all of which means less time and energy to put into weight control."

The Mommy Weight Gain

By their midthirties, many women are having their last children—and increasing numbers are having their first. "Some women feel that during pregnancy, they finally have permission to eat whatever they want," says Robin Kanarek, Ph.D., a physiological psychologist at Tufts University, Medford, Massachusetts. "So they gain too much. If they put on a substantial amount of weight—like 50 to 60 pounds—they may have gained more fat cells, which means it will be much more difficult to take off weight."

And, of course, there's the common phenomenon of being stuck with an extra five pounds after a pregnancy. These five pounds, for reasons that science has yet to fathom, are extremely difficult to lose.

Having borne several children makes it more likely that you've lost and gained weight several times, which brings us to a related problem.

The Yo-Yo Cycle

"Whether weight loss is difficult in the older years depends a lot on how much you've dieted in the past," says weight expert Wayne Callaway, M.D., associate clinical professor of medicine at George Washington University in Washington, D.C. "If I see an older woman, even a postmenopausal woman, who has never dieted, she will do pretty well on a weight-loss program. It's the ones who dieted 40 times who have the most difficulty."

Why? When you lose weight, you lose lots of fat and a little lean muscle. But when you regain, more may come back as fat. It's possible, but not yet proven, that that fat may be harder to get rid of than other fat, and researchers are investigating whether it is more likely to locate itself in the most health-threatening regions: the abdomen and upper body, rather than the safer "below-the-belt" zone on the hips and thighs. Above-the-belt fat has been linked to a higher risk of heart disease and diabetes and may be linked to higher risk of breast and endometrial cancers.

The Empty Nest Syndrome

Older women often face the stress of loneliness when children leave home or because of divorce or widowhood. "Loneliness and too much time on their hands tend to make people eat," says Howard Flaks, M.D., a practicing weight-loss physician in Beverly Hills.

Menopause

Like the midthirties, menopause is another time when there's often a weight spurt. But it's not necessarily the physical fact of menopause that does it, says Rena Wing, Ph.D., a professor of psychiatry at the University of Pittsburgh School of Medicine.

Since 1983, Dr. Wing and her colleagues have conducted the Healthy Women Study. They started the study with 541 healthy premenopausal women aged 42 to 50 years old. Three years later, they studied them again. Many of the women had reached menopause, and the researchers were able to compare them with other women the same age who had not yet reached menopause.

"In general, women tended to gain weight over that period," says Dr. Wing. "But the weight gain occurred in both the 61 women who had a natural menopause by 1987 and the 279 who were still premenopausal." Twenty percent of all the women gained ten pounds or more, and only 3 percent lost ten pounds or more.

"It became clear that the weight gain was an effect of aging, rather than of menopause," concludes Dr. Wing. That doesn't mean weight gain is inevitable: She notes that women who gained the most were those who decreased their activity levels the most, and those who were living alone.

For both the premenopausal and postmenopausal women, weight gain was associated with increases in heart disease risk factors, including blood pressure, total cholesterol level, LDL cholesterol (the bad cholesterol) levels and triglycerides. The women who became menopausal and had the highest weight gain had the most increase in LDL cholesterol.

While menopause itself doesn't cause weight gain, it may well bring an unhealthy shift in the places where fat is stored. Yale biochemist Marielle Rebuffe-Scrive, Ph.D., has found that the activity of a certain kind of enzyme called lipoprotein lipase—which helps attract fat to wherever it resides—declines in the hips and thighs after menopause. Meanwhile, another enzymatic process called lipolysis—which makes it easy to get rid of fat—is reduced in the upper body of postmenopausal women.

Results: After menopause, reduced levels of female sex hormones (estrogen and progesterone) cause more fat to pile on the upper body. That's just what the heart *doesn't* need.

Is Gaining with Age Okay?

Almost every adult gains weight as he or she ages. And we know that excess weight increases health risks. But is this age-related gain really "excess weight"? Is it unhealthy? That's one of the hottest controversies on the medical circuit.

On the one hand, the government's new Dietary Guidelines for Americans, issued in 1990, say that it's acceptable for someone 35 or over to be a little heavier than someone in their twenties as long as (1) the person doesn't have any health condition like diabetes or high blood pressure for which lower weight is required, and (2) the person's fat distribution is more on the hips and thighs than the abdomen. (More fat on the waist puts people at higher risk for diseases like heart disease, diabetes and perhaps breast and endometrial cancer.)

On the other hand, other experts say that the evidence suggests that virtually no weight gain with age is acceptable because of the increased disease risk. These scientists say that until we have better data, we should stick with the old Metropolitan Life Insurance charts, which set weights according to height and frame size and don't allow any weight gain with age.

So what do you do? How do you set weight-loss goals appropriate for you after age 35?

Until there's more research on this important question, there can be no precise answer. But here are some prudent guidelines that may help:

• Since it's possible that there are indeed health risks from having accumulated pounds over what you weighed when you were 19 to 34, it would be smart to play it safe — try to keep your weight close to what it was then. (That is, assuming your earlier weight was within reason.) This is more important if (1) you or your immediate blood relatives have a history of high blood pressure, cardiovascular disease, cancer, diabetes, arthritis or liver disease; (2) your medical examinations show "markers" for these diseases, such as high blood cholesterol levels, high blood pressure and abnormal blood sugar; and (3) you carry most of your excess weight on your stomach, arms or chest instead of your thighs and buttocks.

• But striving mightily to be at this "young" weight is definitely not good if it actually forces you into doing something known to be unhealthy, such as yo-yo dieting, crash dieting, very-low-calorie diets (which can deprive you of nutrients) or trying to accomplish the impossible (and the accompanying stress and misery).

• Weighing the same as you did years ago is not as important to your health as (1) getting 20 to 30 minutes worth of exercise four to six times a week; (2) paring down the fat in your diet to 25 percent of calories or less; and (3) feeling healthy and energetic.

How to Stay Ahead of the Gain

Put on Some Moves

Our experts agree that regular exercise is your number one force for weight control after age 35. It helps you lose unwanted pounds permanently and gives you a big edge in preventing weight gain in the first place. Exercise literally speeds up your metabolism, the rate at which you burn calories. It does this by building muscle, and muscle burns more calories than fat does.

"If you counteract the inevitable decline in metabolism with steady or slowly increased exercise, you'll have more muscle and won't experience decline in calories burned," says Dr. Lowe. What's more, exercise allows older people to eat an adequate amount of food without worrying so much about weight gain.

But increased exercise doesn't mean you should start running marathons, especially if you hate running. "I think that exercise should not be looked upon as doing something until it hurts," says Maria Simonson, Ph.D., Sc.D., director of the Health, Weight and Stress Clinic at the Johns Hopkins Medical Institutions, Baltimore.

The point is to get out there and move. Try walking (a top weight-loss exercise), ballroom dancing, bicycling, rowing, stair climbing, almost anything that gets your limbs moving and your heart pumping a little. High-impact exercises like jogging or high-impact aerobics, though, are not a good idea for 35-plus joints.

New research suggests that strength training can also play a role in speeding up the metabolism and preventing the shift from muscle to fat. After all, strength training builds muscle, your ally in weight loss. "It has to be kept up," says Dr. Lowe. "If you stop, the benefits stop."

"A resistance-training program is good for 35-plus looks, too," says Dr. Blackburn. "If you've lost your muscle tone, it'll help you get it back, and if you do resistance exercise consistently, you won't lose it. Look for a well-supervised program where they have experience with over–35 clients, and talk to your doctor before you start."

You may need to enlist help from family members, perhaps to take on more household chores, to give you extra time for exercise. "The person losing weight with the support and encouragement of family members will do better than the person who tries to do it all on her own," says Dr. Lowe.

If you're over 40, get medical approval before increasing exercise levels or taking on a new form of activity, especially if you have a chronic illness. A doctor might recommend a stress EKG or might be able to tell you if you have osteoporosis, which means you should stay away from high-impact activities. If you have any special injuries, like a bad back, consult an exercise physiologist or physical therapist.

Use Your Maturity

A mature woman brings a lot of resources to the battle of the bulge. "Today's 35-plus woman is getting into her prime," says Dr. Simonson. "She wants her body to reflect that. She knows she'll have to fight a little harder."

Also, a mature woman is probably far less likely than a teenager to swallow a grapefruit diet, a popcorn diet or other gimmicky and unhealthy plans.

Coralie Todd, a travel agent in Los Angeles, California, knows that emotional maturity played an important role in her successful weight loss. At 37, in 1990, she weighed about 390 pounds. But she began losing weight and has dropped 264 pounds since then, on a sensible low-fat diet supervised by Dr. Flaks.

"I always had an obesity problem," says Coralie. "As a young woman I tried all the different diets that are out there, from diet pills to checking into a hospital for a week. I'd lose it and gain it right back. It was a yo-yo situation.

"This diet was different. I felt I had to deal with the issues relating to my obesity. Before I lost the first pound, I worked on my master's degree in psychology. My thesis focused on why I chose to eat. What I was doing for 37 years was hating myself, hating the fat. Until I accepted that it was part of me, I couldn't move on. It was important to love myself, even to love the weight, because in doing that I released the need to have it. A lot of it had to do with self-esteem.

"I didn't do this for the clothes," she adds. "I did this for the health. I was nearing 40 and didn't want the heart disease and all that."

An outlook like Coralie's could help many women. "The idea that extra weight harms health might not carry much impact when you're young," says Dr. Lowe. "But when you get older, the obesity-related health problems are more likely to show up. You feel a sense of responsibility to your family. Your reasons are more profound than just, 'I want to look good for bathing suit season.' "

No More Dieting

Don't think diet; think of making permanent changes in the way you eat. Be sure to eat a low-fat, high-carbohydrate diet and eat meals regularly—not chaotically. "What you eat at 45 should be different from what you ate at 25," says Dr. Simonson. "The older you get, the less food you need without cutting back on nutrients. Of course, you should cut back on fat at any age. Eat smaller portions than when you were younger and take care that the foods you do eat are nutrient dense. Avoid junk foods with few nutrients and many calories. Eat plenty of fruits and vegetables, whole grains, dairy products, fish and lean meats."

To take off pounds, you'll need to combine lower-fat eating with stepped-up exercise. If you try to lose weight by dieting only, you'll lose muscle as well as fat. And less muscle means a slower metabolism. People who eat low-fat diets and exercise regularly are usually more successful at weight loss—and are better able to keep the pounds off. Take it slowly and easily. People over 35 can't expect the same rate of weight reduction as younger people, so be patient. A steady loss of one-half to one pound a week—or slower—is safe.

Don't go below 1,200 calories a day. "Ultralow-calorie diets very, very rarely work long-term," says Dr. Callaway. "From a biological point of view, people on ultralow-calorie diets are starving, and their body sets off adaptive changes, like a slowing of the metabolism, to undermine success." It's also difficult to get the nutrients you need on fewer than 1,200 calories.

There's also an aid to busy weight-watchers that didn't exist in our younger days: prepared low-fat foods such as low-fat frozen dinners, low-fat mayonnaise, even fat-free cheese. "They look like the food you usually eat and enjoy, but the fat has been engineered out, and nutrients have been put in," says Dr. Blackburn.

Before you buy, though, check the label for the answer to these questions.

• Is the food nutrient dense? See that it contains one-third or more of the Recommended Dietary Allowance for several nutrients.
• Is it low in fat? No entrée should contain more than 10 grams of fat, no snack or side dish more than 5 grams per serving.

In testing these kinds of products with clients, Dr. Blackburn has found that women who do use these products improve their chances of successful weight loss by 25 to 30 percent.

Eat Smart in Pregnancy

Again, prevention is the best policy. Talk to your doctor about the appropriate amount of food to eat and weight to gain during your pregnancy. (Losing weight during pregnancy is not recommended.) After pregnancy don't crash diet; take it slowly, sticking with the one-half-to-one-pound-a-week-or-slower rule. "Typically, a lot of women find they can lose almost all the weight they gained during pregnancy, except for maybe an extra five pounds," says Dr. Kanarek. "If it's not more than that, you can live with it. If you get obsessed about it, you may end up with more problems than before."

Counteract a Yo-Yo History

If someone has been dieting for years, successful weight loss may take an even longer amount of time, says Dr. Callaway. "As the first objective, we try to get yo-yo dieters' metabolisms back to normal by giving them a normal amount of calories for their bodies. This is tough at first because they may be used to either starving themselves or gorging themselves."

Clients initially gain weight, Dr. Callaway says, but much of that is water weight. "It may take months for the water weight to come off, so they need a lot of education and support during that time. But I demonstrate to them that it's water by pushing on the shinbone and showing them the dent in the skin that's left." Then it's time for a low-fat diet that's rich in complex carbohydrates and, of course, exercise. The results will show up eventually, on one's figure and the scale.

Reach beyond the Empty Nest

Seek out pleasures and activities unrelated to food if you tend to overeat. "A lot of people who think they want food really want pleasure, solace, comfort and relief from boredom," says Dr. Flaks. "Food is only one of an infinite number of pleasures. I give my clients a list of 150 pleasures: taking a hot bath, calling a friend, getting a pedicure, planning a fantasy vacation. Anything to take their mind off wanting to eat constantly."

If the problems are serious, don't hesitate to get counseling, says Dr. Simonson, who, in her seventies, is still going strong in her profession as a teacher and corporate consultant. "A woman's self-esteem should never go down because she's approaching midlife," says Dr. Simonson.

"Those years can be golden, but you have to work to excavate that gold. You have to know you are a good and worthwhile person and that you can get out there and do things."

Plan Life after Menopause

Anticipate weight gain in the menopausal years and take extra precautions to stay active and not overeat.

One important subject to raise with your doctor is the decision whether to go on hormone replacement therapy (HRT). It's a decision that may have an enormous influence on your weight and your health. You shouldn't base a decision about whether to go on HRT solely on considerations about weight. But HRT's possible effect on your weight is a factor you should put into the equation.

Women who go on hormones gain a little more than those who don't. Much of that weight can be fluid retention, says Dr. Flaks, but the fluid retention can in the long run lead to more fat retention.

It's also very important to note that HRT redirects fat to the lower body regions. So even if you gain a little more weight because of the hormones, it will be in the region where it's less likely to be a health threat.

If you're undecided about hormone replacement, talk to your doctor about the pros and cons.

Yo-Yo Dieting Can Break Your Heart

For some people, trying to stay slim becomes a game of spinning between carrot sticks and cheesecake. Now new research suggests dieters who do the yo-yo—losing and regaining weight repeatedly over time—may actually be toying with their hearts. Researchers found that people with fluctuating weight had a 75 percent higher risk of dying from heart disease than those who maintained a stable weight. These findings were pulled from over 3,000 health records spanning a period of 32 years, as part of the landmark Framingham Heart Study.

"We found that weight variability increased risk, independent of the amount of weight gained," says Dr. Brownell, a coauthor of the study. "Even thin people could be at risk by virtue of many small fluctuations." Not all the facts are in, but yo-yo dieting may prove to be just as tough on your ticker as constant obesity.

Yo-yo dieting may string up your heart by influencing other heart disease risk factors, such as high blood pressure, says Dr. Brownell. "It may also redistribute fat to areas of the body that may lead to a greater risk," he says. Fat may be lost from the thigh, for example, and show up later on a more unhealthy spot like the belly. Even more, people who "weight cycle" may also end up cultivating a stronger preference for fatty foods.

Another study, which looked at women who had been on at least four weight-loss diets in the past year, found that they used up fewer calories during exercise than nondieters. The yo-yoers also weighed more and had more body fat than the nondieters. The researchers suggest that cyclic dieting may cause a dieter to lose lean tissue but gain it back as fat—altering caloric needs.

"If you choose to diet, make sure you're really prepared, and wait for the most optimal conditions to ensure your greatest success," says Dr. Brownell. Eating healthy, with an eye on fruits, vegetables and other low-fat fare, however, should be a lifelong commitment, he adds.

Say Goodbye to Dieting . . . Forever!

What you're about to hear is the final nail going into the coffin lid of the crash diet. A new study—echoing previous research—suggests that as long as you stick to low-fat, delectable fare, you don't have to work to limit the amount of food you eat. You can eat as much as you want—dieting is dead.

Thirteen female volunteers ate either a diet with 37

percent of calories from fat—typical for most Americans—for 11 weeks, or a low-fat diet with no more than 25 percent of calories from fat. The low-fat diet was hardly restrictive: chicken stir-fry, pizza, casseroles and pasta were among the dinners; snacks included ice cream, pudding and cookies. The key was the percentage of calories from fat—all of the meals were under the magic 25. During the low-fat regimen the volunteers lost an average of ½ pound per week—a loss that would amount to 10 percent of one's body weight if stretched over one year. The low-fat eaters ate 220 fewer calories a day than usual and experienced no greater cravings for high-fat foods.

"As long as people eat low-fat versions of the foods they like, they'll lose weight persistently without having to diet," says David Levitsky, Ph.D., professor of nutrition at Cornell University. What's more, if you avoid the padlock-on-the-fridge diet and go the low-fat route, you won't manhandle your metabolism.

"When people diet, their metabolic rate reacts by slowing down," says the researcher. "That's why limiting how much you eat doesn't work in the long run—it decreases your ability to burn calories, and the weight eventually returns." When you feast on low-fat, high-carbohydrate foods without dieting, however, you won't be struck by the bulge boomerang—the weight goes away and stays away.

There are, of course, wonderful long-term benefits of this low-fat fare. Cutting the fat decreases incidence of heart disease and potentially your risk for cancer.

Retire Your Spare Tire

Results of recent studies suggest a strategy that may deflate the midriff monster known as the "spare tire." Here's the plan:

● Limit your alcohol to no more than two drinks a day.
● If you smoke, stop.
● Take a brisk daily walk.
● Load up on complex carbohydrates instead of saturated fat.

According to researchers in California, the belly-busting benefits may be more than cosmetic: "The potbelly has been shown to boost risk for heart disease, diabetes and hypertension," says Elizabeth Barrett-Connor, M.D., professor and chair of the Department of Community and Family Medicine at the University of California, San Diego.

In her study of 1,628 men and women, those who gulped more than two alcoholic drinks a day were found on average to have the largest waist-to-hip ratio, the medical marker for potbelly. There were roughly two times as many large ratios among them as among nondrinkers. Smoking had a similar effect, with two times as many potbellies among puffers as among nonsmokers.

Both exercise and carbohydrate intake seemed to protect against forming the spare tire among men.

This builds on information from another study done in 1987 in which a diet high in saturated fat led to more fat bellies in rats.

Perhaps saturated fats—found in cheesecakes, burgers and cream sauces, for example—have a preference for migrating to the midsection, while carbohydrates—found in vegetables, fruits and grains—lead to a better shape all around.

Sit-ups—even if you do 100 a day—have never been found to melt a potbelly, by the way. They can tone the underlying muscle, but the fat itself does not combust even when your stomach muscles feel like burning coals. The reason: The few minutes it takes to grind out 100 sit-ups aren't nearly enough to torch the fat-burning process. Bouts of brisk aerobic exercise like walking or rowing, lasting 30 minutes or more, are what it takes to ignite fat.

Cutting Fat Takes the Cake

A group of 303 women in their late forties was split into two dietary groups. Some were taught low-fat cooking and food choices and got their diet down to about 21 percent of calories from fat. The rest maintained their usual fat intake of about 39 percent of calories from fat. Neither group restricted overall food or calorie intake, nor were they told to lose weight.

So virtually without trying, the low-fat group lost nearly seven pounds in the first six months—and maintained that lower weight for another six months. Statistically speaking, the women lost a pound for every 3 percent drop in calories from fat.

Researchers say that's because fat in the diet is more easily stored as body fat than protein or carbohydrates, which must be converted to fat. While reducing fat is a good weight-loss strategy, it's not going to be effective if you eat a lot of low-fat but high-calorie alternatives—including sugary sweets.

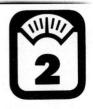

A BEGINNER'S GUIDE TO FIGHTING FAT

Reducing Fat: The Basic Facts

What is today's prime directive of nutrition: Count fat, not calories. Ounce for ounce, dietary fat actually contains more calories (and is more readily converted to body fat) than either protein or carbohydrates. So counting fat automatically counts calories. And we know that a high-fat diet increases our risk of heart disease, cancer and diabetes.

But how do you count fat? And how do you figure out how much is too much for you? Several nutritional authorities recommend that we lower our fat intake so that fat accounts for less than 30 percent of total calories. Other health leaders suggest even lower intakes. (The recipes in Chapter 8 are designed so that no more than 25 percent of calories come from fat.) But is there an easy way to tell when your fat intake is within the guidelines?

The old, standard method was to get out your calculator to figure percentage of calories from fat, either for individual foods or for your whole diet. If you were doing the calculations for foods, you'd have to do some math. First you would check the labels for total grams of fat per serving, then multiply that number by 9, divide by the total calories per serving, and multiply by 100 to get the percentage of calories from fat.

But we're going to show you an easier way that eliminates some of the lengthy calculations. First, check the table on page 21 to find out your "magic number." This is the maximum number of grams of fat you should be eating each day; if your daily intake is under that number, then you're getting no more than 25 percent of your calories from fat and you will be able to maintain your current weight. So all you have to do is count the grams of fat you eat each day and make sure the total doesn't exceed your magic number.

To use the table, find your weight in the first column.

The second column shows the number of calories you're probably eating every day to maintain that weight. The third column is the magic number that you need to memorize.

Let's take the example of a 140-pound woman. The table indicates that to maintain her weight, she's probably eating about 1,680 calories every day. In order to keep her fat intake below 25 percent of calories from fat, she shouldn't eat more than 47 grams of fat a day. And if she wants to *lose* weight, she needs to aim for the fat limit of her goal weight. For example, if the 140-pound woman wants to reduce her weight to 120 pounds, she should

FAT GOALS

For limiting dietary fat to 25 percent of total calories.

Your Weight (lbs.)	Calorie Intake	Fat Limit (g)
Women		♦
110	1,300	37
120	1,400	40
130	1,600	43
140	1,700	47
150	1,800	50
160	1,900	53
170	2,000	57
180	2,200	60
Men		♦
130	1,800	51
140	2,000	54
150	2,100	58
160	2,200	62
170	2,400	66
180	2,500	70
190	2,700	74
200	2,800	78

reduce her fat intake from 47 to about 40 grams of fat per day.

Keep in mind that these fat limits are approximate and that the chart is for sedentary people. If you exercise vigorously, you can afford a little more fat, about 3 grams for every extra 100 calories you burn. The table doesn't account for age, either, and metabolism slows down with age. So it's particularly important for older people to step up their exercise and cut back on fat calories.

To find out how many grams of fat are in the specific foods you eat every day, be sure to check the labels on all packaged foods. You can also refer to the table in Chapter 10.

This approach to counting fat has a way of encouraging some very healthy attitudes toward low-fat eating. With this method, you quickly get used to limiting total fat intake and not fretting about particular foods that contribute to that total. Notice that you don't have to swear off high-fat foods entirely. If you eat small amounts—an occasional pat of butter, a few slices of lean meat—it costs just a few grams of fat. But it's obvious that large amounts of high-fat foods can quickly push you over your fat limit.

This approach also encourages you to eat more of the delicious low-fat alternatives to higher-fat fare. So you'll end up eating more fruits, vegetables, whole grains and other complex carbohydrates while keeping fat intake (and weight) down—which is a good definition of a healthy diet.

5 Steps to Controlling Your Fat Tooth

Once you have figured out your personal fat budget, the trick is to alter your eating habits to meet that budget. Here are some excellent suggestions from Joseph C. Piscatella, author of *Controlling Your Fat Tooth.*

1. Determine Where You Are Now

Now that you know how many grams of fat are in your daily budget, it's time to count up your fat. What are your food preferences right now? And how fat are they? If you could rely on memory, it would be easy to identify frequently eaten fatty foods. But we often forget (or choose to forget) what we eat.

The best way to monitor your present eating habits is to keep a record of your daily food intake. Health professionals usually recommend a three-day record. Simply write down everything you eat during that time. Have a gumdrop? Put it in the record! Be sure to include foods such as salad dressings, butter or margarine and coffee creamer. Keeping a food record may seem like a hassle, but it's the only way to get a look at your real food habits.

It's important not to change anything during this time. Don't start a diet or "be good." Just eat as you normally do, and record everything eaten when it is eaten. By the end of three days, your food record will tell you what and when you eat. It may even give you some insight into why you eat. Most important, it will reveal high-fat habits that need to be changed.

Keep track of your fat intake on the food record and compare it with your budget. (This will not only give you a running total of your fat intake, it will also help you identify favorite foods that are high in fat.) Many food labels provide fat content in grams. Be sure to take "serving size" into consideration. For foods with no nutritional labels, refer to one of the many fat-counting guidebooks on the market.

2. Make Food Palatability a Priority

If experience regarding food behavior has taught us anything, it is this: People will eat healthy, low-fat food only when it tastes good. Most people will not trade taste for health.

Lettuce and carrots may be healthier for us, but they won't offset the craving for a sirloin steak or a wedge of Brie. Better food selection comes about when we shed the concept that healthy food must be boring. Nothing is farther from the truth. A low-fat dietary pattern can involve foods that are tasty, attractive and appealing. The trick is to make low-fat foods so satisfying that high-fat foods are not missed. Would you yearn for prime rib, for example, if you were served hickory-smoked salmon, Cajun turkey breast or seafood fettuccine?

One of the key concepts in fat budgeting is to understand that you can modify your favorite meals without sacrificing taste. Studies show that most American families prepare a dozen recipes 80 percent of the time. The greatest opportunity, then, is to modify these 12 recipes. In doing so, you get the best of both worlds—familiar, favorite foods that conform to your personal fat budget.

3. Learn to Read Food Labels

Fresh, whole foods are the best choices for controlling your personal fat budget. Because of the on-the-run nature of modern life, however, it's unrealistic to think you'll never eat packaged foods. Virtually everyone in the United States, even the most serious antifat activist, at some time eats food from a box or a can. Unfortunately, packaged foods lend themselves to hidden fat, so knowing their fat content is crucial to making informed choices. For this reason, it is essential to know how to read food labels.

Under the present labeling law, nutrition information is required on packaged foods only when a claim is made about nutrition content or when the product is fortified with vitamins, minerals or protein. This covers about 30 percent of foods regulated by the Food and Drug Administration (FDA). Another 30 percent display nutrition information anyway. But that leaves 40 percent with no nutritional data. Some even lack ingredients lists, so we have no clue as to what's in the food. This often means that we end up relying on advertising for information on fat.

Watch out for "low-fat" hype. Food advertising is generally more hype than truthful information. Nowhere is this problem worse than in the promotion of "low-fat" foods. Contrary to advertising claims, many such foods are actually rich in fat. Take ground beef labeled "20 percent fat," for example. It certainly appears to be low in fat, well below the 30 percent guideline. All well and good, except that "20 percent" refers to the weight of fat in the package; that is, fat constitutes 20 percent of total weight. But the body doesn't care what fat weighs. It is more concerned with how many calories fat produces. The truth is that almost 60 percent of calories in ground beef are derived from fat. So, instead of meeting the guideline, it contains about twice the amount of fat recommended.

Many food processors advertise fat content by percentage of weight as a clever way to deceive customers about the true fat content of the product. The information may be technically correct according to the letter of the labeling law, but it certainly violates the spirit. When weight is the measurement used, most foods will look deceptively low in fat. Even hot dogs and sausages can meet this test. Because about half the weight of a hot dog is water, the fat content is just about 30 percent by weight. But fat actually supplies over 80 percent of the calories! This is one reason for using grams of fat in your personal fat budget.

Terms such as *low-fat* and *lean* have little to do with reality. For example, 92 percent of the calories in Kraft Philadelphia Brand Cream Cheese come from fat. It is recognized as a high-fat food. But Kraft Neufchatel Cream Cheese is promoted as a "low-fat" alternative, even though 79 percent of its calories come from fat. How can a food that is four-fifths fat be "low-fat"? It can't! It may be lower in fat than the original product, but it's not low in fat.

4. Count Grams of Fat

The labeling law may undergo changes in the future to give more people access to needed nutritional information. But for now you have to work with labels as they are. Counting grams of fat is the easiest way to use food label information to support your fat-budgeting efforts. This is easily done by referring to the nutritional data on the food label. For example, the following data are found on a carton of whole milk.

Serving size: 1 cup
Servings per container: 4
Calories: 150
Protein: 8 grams
Carbohydrate: 11 grams
Fat: 8 grams
Sodium: 125 milligrams

The label provides two important pieces of information: the number of calories per serving and grams of fat; it shows that a one-cup serving contains 150 calories and 8 grams of fat.

A good rule of thumb is that there should be no more than 3 grams of fat per 100 calories.

Make comparisons of similar products to determine their respective impact on your fat budget. Labels on cheese, for example, show that a one-ounce serving of cheddar has 9 grams of fat, while Parmesan has 7 grams and part-skim mozzarella has just 4 grams.

Or let's assume you'd like a snack and you're eyeing two Hostess Suzy Qs. How much fat is involved? About 20 grams, or almost one-third of your 67-gram fat allotment for the day. A fresh peach, which contains 0.1 gram of fat, would be a better choice. Because of the difference in fat content, the Suzy Qs total 480 calories and the peach just

37. Or put it this way; you could have 13 peaches if you wanted to consume 480 calories. Even if you could eat all 13, they would provide you with less than 2 grams of fat.

It is not that Suzy Qs should be off-limits forever. In a realistic low-fat diet, no single food is forbidden. But if you have a fat budget of 67 grams, and you choose one food with 20 grams of fat, your choices for the rest of the day are very restricted. If you eat something high in fat, balance it out with low-fat foods at other meals to keep within your budget for the day. The trick is not to eat too many high-fat foods.

5. Plan for Change

Your food record will reveal present food habits, and your budget will provide fat and calorie goals. Getting from one to the other means changing food habits. This often seems easy at first. Almost anyone can replace a Danish pastry with an apple—for a week! The challenge is how to make the change stick, to make it a permanent part of your daily life, so that low-fat eating becomes the norm rather than the exception.

It is difficult enough in our fast-paced modern society simply to prepare food, much less to prepare food that is low in fat and also tastes good. If it's 5 P.M. and you're at the store shopping for dinner to be served at 6, you may be too pressed to think of low-fat alternatives. It's very easy then to choose old, familiar, high-fat favorites—hot dogs, frozen meals, fast food. Breaking the high-fat habit is too difficult to accomplish if it's approached in an "as-you-go" fashion. Habits change when you make a plan to change them.

The process of meal planning is really nothing more than preselecting foods that appeal to you and meet your calorie/fat criterion. By planning, you ensure the exclusion of high-fat foods and the inclusion of low-fat ones and min-imize the selections left to chance. Experience shows that if you don't plan ahead to trade your Danish pastry for an apple, it won't happen. There is nothing magical about meal planning; it is simply a tool for success.

Start by examining your food record. It will help you to identify areas that need to be changed. If it indicates you like ice cream as an evening snack, plan to have popcorn instead. You'll still have your snack, so you won't feel deprived, but it will contain less fat and fewer calories.

Plan for reasonable changes; if they're too drastic, you might feel deprived and lose your resolve. If you usually eat a breakfast of bacon and eggs three or four times a week, don't eliminate it from your meal plan. Instead, reduce it to one day a week. Perhaps Saturday could be designated as "bacon and eggs" morning. You can look forward all week to enjoying that special breakfast. Then concentrate on making better breakfast choices for the other six days of the week.

The meal-planning process is easier if you carry a list of foods and meals to choose from. If you're behind schedule when you're shopping for dinner, or you have just a few minutes for a restaurant lunch, you can refer to the list for suggestions.

Meal planning should be realistic and flexible and should reflect your family's tastes and needs. By considering these factors in a plan, you optimize the opportunity to prepare and serve foods that are easy, quick, appetizing and satisfying, yet allow you to stay safely within your fat and calorie budget.

Introducing Fat-Free Foods!

There's a quiet takeover in your local supermarket. Perhaps you haven't even noticed. But, right there, in the

Use These Nonfat Goodies to Your Advantage

All it takes is a little exchange, that's all. No denial, no cravings, no worries. If you use nonfat products to help reduce your dietary fat intake by just 13 grams a day (and that should be easy!), you can lose one pound of body fat in one month. That's without even trying.

And if you cut your fat intake even more (which, with the new nonfat products, isn't too difficult) and get regular moderate exercise (like walking at a brisk pace for about 30 minutes a day), you can lose more than ½ pound a week—easily.

dairy case and packaged-goods aisles, you'll find a mass of new products that have one thing in common: They're fat-free. Go ahead and taste them. Chances are that you, too, will defect from familiar, high-fat prepared foods and join the new fat-free revolution. You're certain to be glad you did.

Good News

Thanks to a little food-processing ingenuity and a growing nutrition-conscious market, you can keep your fat intake in line without giving up the tastes you love! Cookies, frozen desserts, puddings and a multitude of other popular foods have gone lean—really lean.

Think of the positive impact these foods can have on a heart-healthy diet, too. After all, many of the food products that have gone fat-free were originally heavy in butter and cream—both major sources of saturated fat. And research indicates that fat, especially saturated fat (found mainly in animal products), drives up blood cholesterol. That's why lowering the intake of overall fat and saturated fat has been strongly recommended by the National Cholesterol Education Program. It's also why the new fat-free alternatives come as welcome news to anyone who's cholesterol conscious.

Rave Reviews

Here are the new foods our taste-testers loved.

Cookies. Remember Mom's homemade oatmeal cookies? Even today, most recipes call for a stick or two of butter for a batch. Not surprisingly, then, each cookie can ooze with grams of fat, over ½ gram of it saturated fat. Switch to Frookie's fat-free oatmeal-raisin version (which we found to be quite tasty and chewy) and you're in for big fat savings—4 grams for a two-cookie snack.

You can find other varieties of fat-free cookies as well. Health Valley, for example, offers a wide selection of nonfat cookies and fruit bars.

Pudding. Traditional chocolate pudding is a favorite dessert for many people. But, with 6 grams of fat per serving (almost 3½ grams of which are saturated fat), that's a far cry from a light dessert.

Now, however, there's a pudding that's just as delightful and creamy as any pudding you've ever tasted—and (you guessed it) it's fat-free. We taste-tested Jell-O Free Chocolate-Vanilla Swirl Pudding Snacks, available in serving-sized cups in the dairy case. Our pudding aficionados gave it the thumbs-up. The consistency and flavor were as good as original Jell-O Pudding Snacks, they said. Of course, fatwise and caloriewise, the Jell-O Free Pudding Snacks were a hit, too. Compared with the original version, they were 70 calories lighter; compared with homemade, they had about 90 fewer calories.

You can also buy instant pudding mixes in various flavors and make your own fat-free dessert by using skim milk instead of whole milk or low-fat (1 or 2 percent) milk.

Frozen desserts. Simple Pleasures: The name does not deceive you. We sampled this nonfat frozen dairy dessert (in the toffee-crunch flavor) and were delighted with its taste and smooth, creamy consistency. With products like this, you'll never scream for ice cream again! In fact, the only discernible difference we detected was that it did not coat the tongue and linger the way ice cream does. But, hey, when you consider the fat savings (almost 7½ grams of saturated fat and nearly 12 grams of total fat per ½-cup serving) compared with premium vanilla ice cream, you'll agree it's a winning choice.

Many nonfat frozen yogurts have also appeared on the market in recent years, and they are quite delicious. By substituting nonfat vanilla yogurt for a ½-cup serving of premium vanilla ice cream, you save about 12 grams of fat—7½ grams of it saturated—and are spared about 75 calories.

Sour cream. Yikes! Regular sour cream has 3 grams of fat (almost 2 grams of it saturated) in every tablespoon. Thank goodness for fat-free sour creams. Not only do they eliminate the fat, but they are also about 20 calories lighter per tablespoon. Our testers tried Light N' Lively brand and found it satisfying. Nonfat sour cream is a great way to keep Mexican dishes and baked potatoes from becoming cholesterol nightmares. It also holds up well in cooking.

Egg substitutes. The little guys look harmless enough. But eggs contain 5 grams of fat—over 1½ grams of saturated fat—and 75 calories each. Frozen egg substitutes are now available fat-free and have cut two-thirds of the calories from the real McCoy. Although they aren't the newest fat-free foods available, the variety of uses for egg substitutes establishes them as a universal kitchen staple.

Mayonnaise-style dressing. Kraft Free has done it. They have created a terrific nonfat mayonnaise-style dressing. We found that when blended into tuna, chicken or potato salad, it is virtually indistinguishable from the traditional oil-laden versions. Each tablespoon saves you 11 grams of fat, and over 1½ grams of it is saturated fat.

Muffins. Great any time of day, muffins can be a terrific source of fiber. Butter, oil and other high-fat ingredi-

The Secret Ingredient: A Good Whipping

What makes these nonfat versions of foods so similar to their fat-rich ancestors? The answer is, they taste like they have fat in them. That's not done with bizarre and possibly risky new chemicals, either. What does the trick is novel manipulation of many familiar ingredients.

"One fat replacement, Simplesse, is made from proteins that are microparticulated, or beaten into tiny spheres," says Rudolph Harris, Ph.D., consumer safety officer for the Food and Drug Administration (FDA). "These particles are so small that when they are put into a food in place of fat, the product actually has the feel of a fat to the mouth." Simplesse is the fat substitute in Simple Pleasures, the frozen dairy dessert we tested. It is made from microparticulated egg whites and/or milk proteins and other ingredients.

Many of the other fat replacements in fat-free and low-fat products are the result of commercial techniques of acidifying, blending or heating proteins, carbohydrates or fat-based ingredients. Common food ingredients like gums, pectin and starches are used. Other fat replacements that are just as standard as other natural ingredients are dextrin, polydextrose, maltodextrin and cellulose. The innovative use of these elements in foods is recognized as acceptable by the American Dietetic Association. Although the ingredients we've listed above are being used in many nonfat and low-fat foods, the only fat replacement the FDA has approved is Simplesse—and only for its use in frozen desserts. The other ingredients have not yet been tested for use in nonfat or low-fat foods.

ents, however, make many of them undesirable. Mc-
Donald's (yes, the golden arches) has come up with a fat-
free apple-bran muffin that is perfect for people on the go.
A traditional homemade muffin the same size has almost 8
grams of fat and almost 2½ grams of it is saturated fat.

Health Valley has also created a few varieties of fat-
free muffins, available through your supermarket or health-
food store. The muffins come in flavors such as banana,
apple raisin and raisin spice. Compared with a like-size,
traditional bran muffin, a Health Valley fat-free muffin saves
over 5 grams of fat and 1½ grams of saturated fat.

Crackers. Wheat crackers are not high-fat demons if
you eat a modest number of them. Modesty, unfortunately,
is not always snacking policy. At about 60 calories a serving (that's just seven crackers), wheat crackers also deliver
almost 2 grams of fat, 1 gram of it saturated.

Health Valley to the rescue, again. They've come out
with a line of fat-free crackers that are terrific for snacking
with your favorite low-fat and nonfat dips. We really liked
the Organic Wheat with Natural Herbs flavored crackers.
And they have 20 fewer calories and over twice the fiber of
ordinary wheat crackers. Although they were a bit dry
when eaten plain, these crackers had a distinct flavor that
would easily complement salsa or a low-fat bean dip.

Granola bars. This ever-popular snack food is usually only moderately high in fat, although some brands do
contain more as a result of high-fat additions, such as
chocolate chips.

Once again, Health Valley has come up with a palatable fat-free snack. Their granola bar saves you almost 8½
grams of fat (and over 1 gram of saturated) when compared
with an ordinary bar the same size. And let's not overlook
the almost 80 calories you save as well.

Cheeses. Cheeses can be one of the foods people
find most difficult to give up in order to control cholesterol
or lose weight. Whole-milk mozzarella has over 6 grams of
fat, including nearly 4 grams of saturated fat per ounce.

Cheddar is even more trouble, with over 9 grams of total fat and almost 6 grams of saturated fat per ounce.

Thanks to newer fat-free varieties, we can feel good about eating our cheesy favorites again. We tested Alpine Lace Free N' Lean Cheddar to see how it held up against a traditional cheese. Although there was a definite difference in texture and taste, the Alpine Lace was not bad. Melted on top of a piece of toast with a slice of tomato, it was quite good.

The nonfat mozzarella was voted an acceptable alternative to whole-milk mozzarella, too. One tester exclaimed, "I can finally have pizza again!"

Oh, we should also mention that the Alpine Lace nonfat cheddar we tried had about 70 fewer calories than traditional cheddar. That's a big savings in itself.

Cream cheese. Alpine Lace has done it again. Their new Free N' Lean Fat-Free cream cheese and cream-cheese spreads boast a trim 4 percent of calories from fat—compared to ordinary cream cheese with 90 percent fat calories. (Although Free N' Lean isn't completely fat-free, each serving contains less than ½ gram of fat.) You save 10 grams of fat (over 6 grams of it saturated fat) and about 70 calories with every ounce (two tablespoons).

Alpine Lace Free N' Lean Fat Free cream-cheese spreads come in many tempting flavors. You can choose from garlic-and-herb, cheddar, cheddar with jalapeño, and cream-cheese-and-chive flavors. So, spread the news—cream cheese has gone fat-free!

Doubters Should Add It Up

If you're still not convinced that these new foods with no fat can help you lose weight and lower your cholesterol, maybe you should look again. All the new fat-free foods listed in this chapter (which comprise only a fraction of those on the market) add up to nearly 90 grams total fat and almost 40 grams saturated fat *saved* over ordinary foods. Not bad for a bunch of lightweights.

Slash Your Saturated Fat

The new fat-free foods can do more than help you lose weight. They can also help reduce the amount of saturated fat in your diet—and that helps lower your blood cholesterol and your risk of heart disease.

By cutting your saturated fat intake from 20 to 10 grams in an average 1,800-calorie-per-day diet, you can lower your blood cholesterol by ten points in just one month, according to Mark Hegsted, M.D., of the Northeast Regional Primate Center in Southboro, Massachusetts. That's nothing to sneeze at. In fact, reducing your cholesterol by 10 percent could mean you've decreased your chance of developing heart disease by about 20 percent.

7 Master Strokes for Fat Fighting

To maximize the benefits of eating to lose fat, you'll need to make some new habits and break some old ones. Here are five things that you want to avoid, or at least minimize, in your diet:

1. Alcohol. Alcohol is what we call "empty calories"; when you drink you don't get anything nutritious from it. You just get fat and lots of calories.

How many calories? If you have five or six drinks—beers, glasses of wine, mixed drinks—you've racked up 1,000 calories, which is about what people on a healthy diet get from half a day's worth of food. You just can't burn that off.

One drink a day? A beer after work or a glass of wine with dinner is fine. You don't have to abstain completely. Just remember, you're drinking calories.

2. Fast foods. Very high in fat and calories. Again, you just can't exercise this much fat off. Sure, it tastes good, but it's just not worth the amount of fat that you're putting in your body. And fast-food places are disasters for people trying to cut down on salt. You get a week's worth of salt in one meal.

3. Condiments. Butter, salad dressing, mayonnaise—lots of fat here. Often, when you add condiments to a meal, you're adding more fat to what you're eating than there was to begin with.

The worst? Salad dressing. If you think you just can't eat a salad without a little bit, at least ask for it on the side. Don't ever let anybody put it on the salad for you. Just pour some flavored vinegar on top if you want a little extra taste. You don't need the oil.

4. Late-night eating. The worst food you eat is after 9 or 10 P.M. And the killer is that you're probably not even hungry—just bored. It's emotional. You're just eating to eat.

If you're really hungry at night, try eating better during the day. Eat a bigger, healthy lunch later in the day and then eat dinner later. If you have to eat something late, have some bran cereal with fruit and low-fat (1 percent) or skim milk. And then take a walk.

5. Traditional dining out. You can't eat out four or five times a week and not get fat. No matter how carefully you order, it just can't be done.

That's what to avoid. Now here's what avoiding them will do for you, in combination with the kind of fat-burning exercise program described in Chapter 4.

By eliminating or greatly reducing any one, you'll stop gaining weight.

Eliminate two and you'll lose a little weight and you'll

start changing your body composition. You'll start to shape up a little.

With three, you're heading toward your ideal body composition. Most of the weight loss will be the fat you hate the most. People will start to tell you that you look better.

Avoid four for long enough, and you will attain your ideal body composition. That may not mean that you'll look like a picture in a magazine swimsuit ad, but keep in mind that that may be an unrealistic goal, because that person is not you. It means that you'll look as good as you possibly can given your height, basic build, bone structure and genetic makeup.

You'll also improve your overall health and well-being. And without a doubt, you'll feel better.

While you're changing your habits, here are two positive habits to adopt as integral parts of your new eating behavior:

1. Fruit and vegetables. Eat fruit every day. Make sure you get four or five servings of fruit or vegetables daily. Not only are they good for you, they also replace other foods that aren't.

2. Fiber. Get lots of fiber from whole grains and whole-grain cereals and breads. It's great stuff and it fills you up. You can't be hungry after you eat fiber-rich foods.

Cooking Light: Test Your "Lean-Literacy"

It's not easy to keep up with all you need to know about healthy cooking. In fact, some of the basic skills probably wouldn't be in any health-conscious cook's repertoire—things like baking with chocolate or making gravy.

But now that you are starting to think about what techniques a cook concerned with fat-cutting, fiber-adding and nutrient-preserving should know, it's a perfect time to learn. This test, designed by Diane Drabinsky, a registered dietitian, will let you test your knowledge of healthy modern cooking.

1. Which milk is lowest in fat?
   a. 1% milk
   b. 2% milk
   c. Whole milk
   d. Evaporated skim milk
   e. Don't know

2. What is a quick method for preparing dried beans?
   a. Soak beans overnight in three to four times their volume of water. Drain. Cover again with water and simmer until soft.
   b. Buy canned beans.
   c. Cover beans in three to four times their volume of water. Bring to a boil. Remove from heat, cover tightly and let sit for two hours. Drain, cover again with water and simmer until soft.
   d. Place beans in baking dish, cover with water and bake for one hour.
   e. Don't know.

3. When cooking rice or other grains you use _____ as much water as the grain you are cooking.
   a. Three times
   b. Four times
   c. Twice
   d. Don't know

4. An appropriate no-cholesterol egg substitute for one large egg would be:
 a. Two egg whites
 b. Two egg whites plus half a yolk
 c. One cup of commercial egg substitute
 d. Don't know

5. Low-fat yogurt can be all or partially substituted for the following ingredients in most recipes:
 a. Sour cream
 b. Mayonnaise
 c. Whipped cream
 d. All of the above
 e. Don't know

6. Which cooking method(s) will best retain the vitamin and mineral content of vegetables?
 a. Microwaving
 b. Boiling
 c. Steaming
 d. Frying
 e. A and C
 f. Don't know

7. A lean cut of meat will:
 a. Have very little marbling and excess fat
 b. Be very red
 c. Come from a very soft part of the animal
 d. Be sliced very thin
 e. Don't know

8. A high-fat fish like salmon can still be part of a heart-healthy diet.
 a. True
 b. False
 c. Don't know

9. To remove the fat from meat drippings you can:
   a. Strain it
   b. Refrigerate it
   c. Boil it
   d. Thicken it
   e. Don't know

10. A heart-healthy portion of cooked meat is:
   a. 5 ounces
   b. 4 ounces
   c. 3 ounces
   d. 6 ounces
   e. Don't know

11. The best method for separating an egg is:
   a. Passing the yolk back and forth between the two eggshell halves while the egg white falls into a dish
   b. Use an egg separator
   c. Break an egg into a dish and scoop the yolk out with a spoon
   d. Don't know

12. When sautéing vegetables you can use water, stock and/or wine in place of the oil.
   a. True
   b. False
   c. Don't know

13. A substitute for buttermilk would be:
   a. Half-and-half
   b. Evaporated milk
   c. Milk and vinegar
   d. Milk and baking soda
   e. Don't know

14. Where is most of the fat found on poultry?
   a. The wings
   b. Deposited between the breast and legs
   c. The skin
   d. Don't know

15. Many hard cheeses like cheddar are low in fat and can be used liberally in recipes.
   a. True
   b. False
   c. Don't know

16. To increase the fiber content of baked products you can successfully substitute _____ the amount of white flour with whole-wheat flour.
   a. One-quarter
   b. Half
   c. Two-thirds
   d. Don't know

17. To obtain a 3-ounce portion of cooked meat you start with _____ ounces of raw meat.
   a. 5 ounces
   b. 6 ounces
   c. 4 ounces
   d. Don't know

18. Three lean cuts of beef are:
   a. Top round, tenderloin and round tip
   b. Rib, top round and top loin
   c. Top round, chuck and sirloin
   d. Don't know

19. Low-fat cooking methods include:
   a. Baking, frying and sautéing
   b. Grilling, broiling and frying
   c. Broiling, grilling and sautéing
   d. Don't know

20. The ingredient in marinades that will tenderize less tender cuts of meat is:
   a. The acid (vinegar)
   b. The herbs and spices
   c. The fat (oil)
   d. Don't know

21. Your recipe calls for one tablespoon of fresh parsley but you only have dried. You would use _____ dried parsley.
   a. Two teaspoons
   b. ½ teaspoon
   c. One teaspoon
   d. Don't know

22. Salt must always be added to a recipe if called for.
   a. True
   b. False
   c. Don't know

23. When pasta is cooked correctly there is no need to add butter or margarine to avoid sticking.
   a. True
   b. False
   c. Don't know

24. White rice, brown rice, millet, bulgur, barley and oats are all whole grains.
   a. True
   b. False
   c. Don't know

Answers

1. (a) Evaporated skim has less than ½ gram of fat per ½ cup.

2. (c) You can used canned beans, but rinse off the sodium first.

3. (c)

4. (a) One cup of substitute is enough to replace four eggs.

5. (d) Low-fat yogurt can be substituted for all of the ingredients listed.

6. (a) and (c)

7. (a) Marbling is fat.

8. (a) Much of the fat is heart-healthy omega-3s.

9. (b)

10. (c)

11. (b) A separator minimizes the danger of bacterial contamination from the shell.

12. (a) For a buttery flavor without fat, add some butter-substitute granules.

13. (c)

14. (c)

15. (b) But some high-fat cheeses have strong enough flavor to be used sparingly.

16. (b)

17. (c)

18. (a)

19. (c) All can be done without adding fat.

20. (a)

21. (c) Drying concentrates the flavor of herbs, so you use less dry than fresh.

22. (b)

23. (a)

24. (b) White rice is not a whole grain; the rest are.

Scoring

Give yourself one point for every right answer, and zero points for every one you got wrong or answered "Don't know."

Under 17: Maybe you should consider some cooking lessons.

17–20: Keep up the good work. You're on the way to becoming a really healthy cook.

21–23: You're in very good shape, cooking wise, and well above average.

24: Congratulations! You're an M.H.C. (Master of Healthy Cooking).

Foods of the Future
By Mary Hubbard, R.D., Ph.D.

If someone who died ten years ago (better make that five years ago) came back to life and visited a local supermarket, many of the food products being sold today would be unrecognizable. Our growing concern for slim, healthy bodies has prompted research and development into "future foods." Of course, some of the more promising foods of the future include artificial sweeteners and artificial fats. Food science is constantly working on ways to let us have our cake (chocolate with creamy frosting, of course) and eat it, too.

Sweeteners

Everyone is familiar with the incredible success of NutraSweet brand sugar substitute. After the concerns about saccharin were aired (a Canadian study suggested that saccharin caused malignant bladder tumors in rats that were fed huge amounts of the substance, although current evidence is building again to support saccharin's

safety), consumers were primed and ready for a new sweetener. NutraSweet filled the gap. Its great success spurred
investigation into other sweeteners, especially ones that
could be used in cooking. NutraSweet has the drawback of
losing its sweetening ability if used at sustained high temperatures. So the search for the perfect sugar substitute is
still on. The following are some of the new and future en-
tries in the battle for America's sweet tooth.

Alatame

Pfizer, Inc., has submitted a petition to the FDA for the
approval of its sweetener, alatame. It is 2,000 times sweeter
than sugar and is formed from two amino acids (the building blocks of protein), just as is aspartame (the chemical
name of NutraSweet). It is reportedly more stable than aspartame and may thus be used in baked goods as well as
beverages.

Sucralose

A subsidiary of Johnson and Johnson, McNeil Spe-
cialty Products Co., has submitted a petition to the FDA for
approval of a sweetener that is made from sugar but is 600
times sweeter. Because it is made from sugar it has excellent stability even at high temperatures, so it is suitable for
use in a broad range of foods, including beverages, baked
goods, chewing gum, dairy products (like ice cream), sy-
rups and even tabletop sweeteners you use to sweeten your
coffee or cereal.

Left-Handed Sugar

The perfect sugar substitute probably doesn't exist,
but left-handed sugar (L-sugar for short) sounds very close.
This is a substance with its molecules arranged in the mirror image (much as your left hand is the mirror image of
your right hand) of regular sugar. The big difference is, it
can't be digested and absorbed by your body because our

digestive systems only "fit" the regular sugar arrangement. It would be like trying to put your left hand into your right glove. And if it can't be digested and absorbed, it will pass right through the body so it can't supply any calories. L-sugar supposedly looks like, cooks like, and most important, tastes like regular sugar.

Fats

Now the artificial fats enter into the picture. Fat of all kinds (solid, liquid, saturated or unsaturated) is a concentrated form of calories. Fat provides nine calories in only 1 gram (about the weight of a small paper clip), whereas protein or carbohydrate each provide four calories per gram. And evidence is building that dietary fat is more easily converted to body fat than are either carbohydrate or protein. So if we could find a way to decrease the fat in our diets (without making any sacrifices, of course), then we could reduce our calories even more drastically than by using sugar substitutes. Imagine fat-free french fries and rich ice cream with less than half the calories.

Simplesse

This artificial fat is claimed by the NutraSweet Co. to be the first and only all-natural fat substitute. Simplesse is made by cooking and blending milk and/or egg white protein to make a creamy fluid with a texture so like fat it fools the tongue. It is completely digestible but substitutes one or two calories of protein for nine calories of fat. Total calorie savings in products will range from 20 to 80 percent.

Simplesse has some limitations, however. Frying or baking will cause Simplesse to gel and lose its creaminess, which limits its uses. Simplesse will probably not be sold for home use but will be sold to food manufacturers as an ingredient in sour cream, cream cheese, margarine, yogurt and ice cream.

Simplesse has already received approval by the FDA.

In fact, Simple Pleasures ice cream, which utilizes Simplesse, is currently making its way across America. Its level of acceptance will determine if more products using Simplesse are in our future. One attractive possibility is the combination of Simplesse and NutraSweet in the same product, a creamy sweet frosting, perhaps? After all, the NutraSweet Co. owns the patent on both.

Olestra

Procter and Gamble has been researching "olestra," a fat substitute made from sugar and vegetable oil. This substance is calorie-free because it is not digested or absorbed by the body. Research shows olestra may lower the absorption of cholesterol from food in our digestive systems. This is a definite health bonus, but one that has caused the FDA to demand that even more intensive research be conducted on its safety before it can be approved. Using 100 percent olestra for a cooking oil is not feasible, as it causes diarrhea, so it is blended about 50–50 with regular cooking oil. It is said to look, cook and taste like regular oils. It is not broken down by cooking temperatures and can be used in baked goods, fried snacks and frozen desserts.

As revolutionary as these new products are, we need to put these possibilities into perspective. Studies have shown that even with the availability of artificial sweeteners (and Americans are guzzling millions of cans of sugar-free soft drinks each year), we have not really reduced our overall caloric intake. It seems we just eat more of other things to make up for the ones we have given up. So remember, a healthy, nutritious and, yes, delicious diet is not a function of any individual food or product like artificial sweetener or artificial fat. It is determined by a diet rich in a variety of fruits, vegetables, whole grains, lean meats and low-fat dairy products.

Reprinted with permission from *American Fitness* magazine, November/December 1991.

The Quest for the Best Cookie

Cookie makers these days are devilishly good at working both sides of the aisle. On the one hand, they try awfully hard to convince us that their sweet treats are good for us by adding oat bran, substituting honey or fruit juice for sugar and dropping tropical oils from their recipes. But these ploys rarely lower the fat and calorie numbers much, if at all.

On the other hand, they tempt us—often successfully—with rich, cream-filled and chocolate-slathered new cookies that have fat and calorie profiles that rival candy bars.

It's enough to make you think there can't possibly be any place for cookies in a healthy diet.

Good news—there is. All you need to do is read the labels to identify your best cookie choices. Look for those that get 30 percent of their calories, or less, from fat. To put it another way, that's 3 grams of fat, or less, for every 100 calories.

Keep an eye on the actual grams of fat, too. In a few cases, like Pepperidge Farm's Linzer cookie, the calories are so high (120 in one cookie) that even a whopping 4 grams of fat only comes to 30 percent of calories from fat. But indulge in just two of those sweet diet bombs and you've used up 8 grams of your fat budget—almost one-fifth of your daily 44-gram allotment if you are a 130-pound woman!

And as you'll find from reading labels, there are plenty of cookies with even more grams of fat—the undisputed champ being the Oreo Big Stuff, stuffed with 12 grams of fat and 250 calories in one cookie. Somehow it's no surprise to learn that there is lard in them, too.

A cookie that is slightly higher than 30 percent of calories from fat can redeem itself somewhat if it has ingredients like bran, whole wheat or oats or a fairly high-fiber fruit like figs or raisins. (Don't even think about counting that as a serving of fruit, though!) If those foods are close to the top of the ingredients list on the package, they probably contribute some nutrients.

But even healthy ingredients won't salvage some diet disasters, like Pepperidge Farm's Irish Oatmeal cookies with 5 grams of fat (50 percent of calories) in ½ ounce.

In fact, Pepperidge Farm and Nabisco both offer tasty alternatives that are lower in fat, so why choose those that are padded with it?

Little Cookie—Big, Bad Surprise

The latest success story in cookies is miniversions of regular-sized standbys. They're supposed to offer a smaller serving to health-conscious consumers, but beware—for some unknown reason, some of the miniversions have more fat than their regular-sized cousins. A case in point: Nabisco's Apple Cinnamon Graham Bites have 2 grams of fat per ½ ounce, which is 30 percent of their calories, while the full-sized Cinnamon Grahams have only 1 gram of fat that contributes 15 percent of the calories.

Likewise, one regular Pecan Sandie has 80 calories and 5 grams of fat, but four bite-sized Pecan Sandies have 90 calories and 5 grams. Who's going to stop at four?

Another problem with minicookies is that their size makes it even easier to scarf several handfuls mindlessly. Eleven Teddy Grahams have 60 calories and only 2 grams of fat, but who really counts? You can pop them in your mouth by the handful. (Some kids we know put away Teddy Grahams by the bowlful!)

So unless you can ration yourself, it might be best to stick with regular-sized cookies.

Tips for Avoiding a Chocolate Mess

Though most cookies are now made with vegetable oil, you'll still find lard lurking in some, cleverly disguised as "animal shortening" on the label. This is bad news for chocolate lovers, since lard appears mostly in fudge and chocolate cookies. Although you don't get a lot of cholesterol from the lard in these cookies—in most it's about 2 milligrams per cookie—you certainly don't need it. And if you really have to watch your cholesterol intake, you'd best cross such cookies off your list permanently.

But if you absolutely must have chocolate, try Nabisco's Chocolate Snaps with 2 grams of fat in four cookies (26 percent of calories), or their Devil Food Cakes with 1 gram of fat (13 percent). Both are made with vegetable shortening.

Here are a few other pointers for chocolate fans:

• Avoid fancy chocolate names and chocolate-nut combinations. For example, Pepperidge Farm's Beacon Hill Chocolate Chocolate Walnut, Chesapeake Chocolate Chunk Pecan or Sausalito Milk Chocolate Macadamia all have 120 calories per one-ounce cookie and 7 grams of fat (53 percent).
• Nabisco's Chocolate Chocolate Chunk weighs in at 90 calories and 5 grams of fat per ½-ounce cookie, and their Chocolate Chunk Pecan at 100 calories and 6 grams of fat.

Let's face it, any cookie that has the word *chocolate* in its name twice, or words like *chunk* or *double*, probably isn't a good choice.

The Low-Fat Lineup

So far, we've told you what to avoid on the cookie aisle. Now here are some suggestions for selecting cookies that can fit into a healthy diet.

● Pepperidge Farm's new line of Wholesome Choice Cookies are delicious, low-fat choices for that occasional snack.
● Other low-fat choices include R. W. Frookie, Weight Watchers and Health Valley sweets.
● If you enjoy simple vanilla wafers, your best bet are Nabisco's Nilla Wafers. You can snack on 3½ cookies for only 60 calories and 2 grams of fat.

Consider these low-fat, and sometimes nonfat, alternatives to cookies: sweetened minirice cakes (like Hain's Honey Nut and Chico San's Apple Cinnamon), cinnamon and sugar graham crackers and animal crackers, and cinnamon-raisin minibagels.

Of course, the way to be sure you've got a low-fat cookie is to bake it yourself.

Look What They've Done to My Oreos

Everybody's favorite childhood cookie, regular Oreos have 50 calories and 2 grams of fat (36 percent)—not bad in small quantities. But in the name of brand extension, Nabisco added more of the white filling in the middle. That jumps Oreo Double Stufs to double the fat—4 grams—and 51 percent of calories. And then they created a monster: Oreo Big Stuf, which at 1¾ ounces per cookie, packs an enormous 250 calories and 12 grams of fat!

Here's yet another reason to stick to the classic original: Oreos covered in fudge or white fudge have more than double the calories and three times the fat.

When you're figuring out your fat budget for the day, remember this—one Oreo Big Stuf equals four Fig Newtons for calories and twelve Fig Newtons for fat content!

Move Over, Ice Cream:
The New Frozen Yogurts Are Hot!

In less than 20 years, yogurt has shed its earth-shoes-and-bean-sprouts aura and now threatens to replace ice cream—our all-time favorite food—in the hearts and mouths of Americans. While ice cream sales remained flat in the late 1980s, sales of frozen yogurt nearly doubled.

But is frozen yogurt really a better choice than ice cream? Yes! But it's not because of something magical in the bacteria that turn milk into yogurt. Many researchers are not yet convinced that the bacteria (yes, that means germs, but these are good germs) that make yogurt yogurt really have any impact on your health. All those stories about rugged, long-lived yogurt-eating mountain men in the Caucasus may be just that—stories.

And the healthfulness of any given frozen yogurt is not guaranteed. Right now, one product labeled "frozen yogurt" may have a lot more fat and a lot less yogurt in it than another one that says the same thing. It may even have as much fat as some ice creams.

That's because the demand for frozen yogurt has grown more quickly than the federal government has been able to set standards for the product. Current regulations say ice cream must have a certain amount of fat in it. But yogurt rules, when they arrive, will probably limit the amount of fat in frozen yogurt that calls itself "low-fat" and set certain levels for active yogurt cultures and acidity.

Until the government decides what can be called "low-fat" or "nonfat" frozen yogurt, you'll have to read labels carefully. We'll tell you what to look for.

A Good Bet for Less Fat

While the scientific jury is still out on yogurt as a great boon to health, there's not a whole lot of question that most of the frozen yogurts on the market are much lower in fat than most ice creams. And a panel of taste-testers— devoted ice cream fans all—found a number of brands that are as sweet, creamy and satisfying as most ice creams.

But at least a few of these products aren't much lower in fat and calories than ordinary supermarket ice cream. Some frozen yogurt makers get around that by giving numbers for a three-ounce serving, while the ice cream information is for four ounces.

By working out the fat and calories for only one ounce, you can figure out if someone is trying to fool you. A frozen yogurt that has 100 calories and 3 grams of fat in a three-ounce serving comes in at 33 calories and 1 gram of fat per ounce—not much different from an ice cream that has 120 calories and 4 grams of fat in four ounces.

When you're reading labels, look for a frozen yogurt that has 1 gram of fat or less per ounce. That should be easy, since many brands have absolutely no fat. Fat levels don't appear to have that much impact on the texture or taste of many brands, going by the opinions of our tasters. They loved Häagen Dazs' vanilla almond crunch, which had the highest fat level of the yogurts. But most of them liked Kemp's nonfat version nearly as much.

Looking for the Lactobacillus

How do you know if what you're buying is really frozen yogurt or an ice cream clone? "If it says 'Contains live yogurt cultures,' the predominant ingredient is most likely active yogurt," says Manfred Kroger, Ph.D., a professor of food science at Pennsylvania State University and one of America's most respected authorities on dairy products. "Otherwise, if 'cultured milk' is well down on the ingredients list, it probably doesn't have many bacteria in it."

Dr. Kroger feels that federal standards for frozen yogurt are less than a year away. "One thing they must set is a standard for live yogurt cultures in a frozen yogurt. The cultures set up a certain amount of acidity, which makes the characteristic sour yogurt flavor," he says. "The manufacturers don't want a really sour flavor, only slightly sour. But to my mind, if you want to cash in on the yogurt name, it has to be sour. If there's no bacteria in it, it shouldn't be called yogurt."

Is Frozen Yogurt Dead Yogurt?

That's a question most people ask about frozen yogurt. "Freezing doesn't automatically inactivate the bacteria that change milk to yogurt," says Manfred Kroger, Ph.D., a professor of food science at Pennsylvania State University. "It depends on a lot of things, beginning with the size of the bacteria population in the yogurt and the freshness of the product. Any yogurt culture, frozen or not, dies over time. So a product can't sit around for a long time and still have active cultures.

"After several weeks of storage, the levels of live bacteria begin to go down," says Dr. Kroger. "Then a large percentage, maybe as much as 80 percent, of that is killed in the stomach during digestion, which doesn't leave much to culture in the intestines. So you can see the importance of having a good-sized live culture in the product to begin with, if it is going to do any good at all."

Dr. Kroger is one of the scientists waiting and working to find out if eating yogurt and other cultured milk products actively improves health—apart from providing a low-fat alternative to ice cream and apart from letting people who are lactose intolerant enjoy dairy products.

"The evidence is mostly anecdotal and theoretical," he says. "There's a theory that these benign bacteria crowd out the undesirable kind in the gut. This may build immunity to germs that cause illness. But it's still only a theory."

Theory or not, Dr. Kroger himself eats yogurt—and drinks cultured sweet acidophilus milk—every day.

Making Your Own Frozen Yogurt

One way to be sure that your frozen yogurt is fresh, has active cultures and is really low in fat or even fat free is to make your own. Simply taking a container of commercial yogurt and putting it in the freezer doesn't work very well. It gets hard and starts to separate once it melts.

But Gail Damerow, author of *Ice Cream! The Whole Scoop*, says it's easy to make rich, creamy frozen yogurt with an ice cream maker, which keeps the yogurt stirred up and blended while it freezes.

Damerow, who owns her own small dairy, is not only an ice cream expert, she's also an ice cream fanatic. Her book is an exhaustive but enthusiastic exploration of the whole world of frozen delights, and she devotes an entire chapter to do-it-yourself frozen yogurt.

Purists like her, she admits, start by making their own yogurt. But those of us with less time (and no cow out back) can use any commercial brand of plain low-fat or nonfat yogurt. For extra creaminess, she suggests adding some undiluted evaporated milk or powdered milk made with only half the usual amount of water.

Here's a sample of her frozen yogurt recipes. We chose some of her lower-fat concoctions, but this is only a small taste of the recipes for frozen treats—ranging from nonfat ices to sinfully rich ice creams—found in her book.

In these recipes, you have several options. You can use heavy cream for greater richness. But light cream, half-and-half or even nonfat evaporated milk will do. But as Damerow points out, you'll trade creaminess and some flavor for reduced calories and fat.

Vanilla Frozen Yogurt

If you're among those who feel that vanilla and yogurt don't mix but that yogurt and honey were meant to be, substitute ½ cup honey for the sugar and ½ teaspoon almond extract for the vanilla and make honey almond frozen yogurt.

> 2 cups plain yogurt
> 1 cup cream
> ⅔ cup sugar
> 2 teaspoons vanilla

Beat the ingredients together until smooth. Chill and stir-freeze.

Makes 1 quart.

Fruity Frozen Yogurt

From vanilla to fruit-flavored frozen yogurt is an easy step. Simply omit vanilla and in place of cream, add puréed berries, banana or papaya sprinkled with 2 tablespoons lemon or lime juice. If you use sweetened canned or thawed frozen fruit, reduce the sugar accordingly.

> 1 cup coarsely puréed fruit
> ⅔ cup sugar
> 2½ cups plain yogurt

Combine the puréed fruit and sugar, beat smooth and blend in the yogurt. Chill and stir-freeze.

Makes 1 quart.

Coffee Frozen Yogurt

For added crunch, include ½ cup of finely chopped toasted almonds. If you want to avoid using whole eggs, use only the whites, whipped to soft peaks. Add them to the chilled mixture while it is freezing.

    ¾ cup sugar
    1 tablespoon instant coffee
    2 cups milk
    2 beaten eggs (or 2 egg whites)
    1 cup plain yogurt
    ½ teaspoon vanilla

In a double boiler, combine the sugar, instant coffee and milk. Heat, stirring until the sugar dissolves. Pour a little of the warm milk into the eggs, then add the egg mixture to the rest of the milk. Heat, stirring, until slightly thickened. Let cool. Then beat smooth and stir in the yogurt and vanilla. Chill and stir freeze.

Makes 1 quart.

Spicy Peach Frozen Yogurt

When you can't wait until peaches are in season, use canned ones and reduce the sugar to ½ cup. This recipe makes a terrific pie filling.

½ cup peaches, peeled and chopped
⅔ cup sugar
3 cups yogurt
⅛ teaspoon nutmeg
¼ teaspoon cinnamon
⅛ teaspoon cloves
1 teaspoon vanilla

Combine the peaches and sugar and set aside for several hours. Beat smooth and stir in the yogurt; beat smooth again and add the spices. Chill and stir-freeze.

Makes 1 quart.

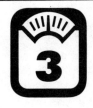

THE NEW NUTRITION: EATING FOR LIFELONG WEIGHT CONTROL

A Shopper's Guide to the New Foods

Remember the days when a typical shopper's basket might contain milk, eggs and a couple of shades of Jell-O? Peek into today's shopper's basket, and you might also spot a carambola and a couple of jicamas.

Supermarkets are exploding! It's the kind of explosion that comes from the arrival of literally thousands of new products every year. The trend began in the 1980s and has gone ballistic ever since.

According to the Food Marketing Institute (FMI), an association that represents supermarket retailers, the number of items carried by a typical supermarket has more than doubled in a decade—from 14,145 in 1981 to 30,000 in 1990. Growth continued through 1991.

What's behind it? Ethnic diversity and our adventurous taste for international cuisine are two driving forces. Once obscure Asian, Latin and European delights are becoming commonplace on supermarket shelves. Technology is another important agent of change. Mother never fed us Broccoflower because it wasn't created yet.

One of the most important influences is our new health awareness. In a 1991 FMI survey, 97 percent of shoppers said nutrition is an important factor when they purchase food. Only taste ranked higher. That's why there's a plethora of new low-fat, high-nutrient products arriving all the time. But food producers know that newly introduced foods must taste great for consumers to bite.

It was with nutrition and fantastic flavor in mind that *Prevention* editors took to the supermarket aisles across the country to find the most exciting, most delicious, healthiest, low-fat, new items available.

Shoppers heard our cries of, "What's this?" echo down the aisles as we pinched and pondered turkey thigh steaks, star fruits, dried morels and sweet-dumpling squash.

Then we talked to the experts about how to best prepare them to enhance their star qualities. We guarantee these foods will fill your meals with flavor—but not fat.

Depending on your own ethnic background and what part of the country you live in, some of these products may not seem so exotic. Corn tortillas are old hat in suburban Los Angeles, but they're a relatively new innovation in suburban Boston. Italian Americans won't blink at broccoli rabe, but the rest of us will (especially after we taste it).

Just a few years ago, most of these foods were considered too exotic, ethnic or gourmet for supermarkets.

Don't despair if you can't find all of these items in your regular supermarket; just try another market. With so many choices, shopping's no longer a chore—it's an adventure!

Aromatic Rice

Now that aromatics have arrived in supermarkets, the brown-rice "blahs" need never strike again. Moments after cooking begins, the kitchen fills with the fragrance of roasted nuts. And aromatic rices don't contain any more fat or calories than regular brown rice.

There are several aromatic brown rices now available. Each offers different textures, though the flavors are all similar—like basmati rice, the granddaddy aromatic that hails from India.

The aroma, incidentally, is not manmade; it's a byproduct of natural compounds found in all rice but present in higher quantities in aromatics.

Buying Tips

Look for words like "aromatic" or "American basmati" on the label. There are three kinds of aromatic rice: basmati (imported from India or Pakistan), American basmati (grown here) and Jasmine (grown in Thailand and the United States). Brown and white varieties are available.

Serving Ideas

● For pilafs and salads, it's best to choose an imported or American basmati. Both cook up like long-grain rice, with separate kernels. (The American basmati is equally fluffy.)

● For a risotto, you need a soft, sticky rice. That's how Jasmine rice cooks up. Jasmine types are available from a few manufacturers in brown-rice varieties.

● To preserve its delicate flavor and aroma, don't overwhelm aromatic rice with strong flavors or thick sauces. Enhance the natural flavor by adding a few roasted nuts or sunflower seeds, fennel seeds, sautéed onions, peas or a bit of saffron.

● Another way to heighten flavor: Before cooking, sauté kernels in a dry pan, stirring constantly, until they start to brown slightly and snap.

Arugula

How good can a leafy green vegetable taste? The ultimate answer: arugula (otherwise known as roquette, rocket, rucolo). Different flavors unfold as you chew—toasted sesame seeds . . . mustard . . . roasted walnuts . . . black pepper . . . hot pepper . . . grilled beef. It's an experience. In the opulent 1980s, this hitherto obscure Mediterranean leaf achieved fame in the United States in trendy restaurant salads.

In the no-frills 1990s, neat bundles of arugula—looking like small, well-ironed spinach or dandelion leaves—can be found for a reasonable price in the produce section of supermarkets across the country. Arugula is a good source of vitamin C (20 milligrams per cup, about 33 percent of the RDA). It's virtually fat-free and has a meager five calories per cup.

Buying Tips

Choose leaves that are a healthy dark green, smooth and free of brown spots, not limp, wilted or yellowed.

Serving Ideas

● Punctuate green salads with arugula, or, when you've grown to adore the stuff, make a salad with arugula as the only green.
● Use it, dressed with a splash of balsamic vinegar, as a bed for grilled lean meats, like beef tenderloin or turkey. It's divine in a sandwich, too.
● Add it to defatted chicken broth, along with garlic, basil and leeks, for an unusual and tasty soup stock.
● Steam or stir-fry it briefly, as you would spinach.

Balsamic Vinegar

Ten years ago you practically had to be an heiress to get hold of a good bottle of balsamic vinegar. It was sold almost exclusively in gourmet stores—and even then, diligent searching was required. Aged in wooden barrels, a four-ounce jar of the precious brown fluid could set the trust fund back by $100.

But over the past five years balsamic vinegar has become America's favorite flavored vinegar, and a sizable good-quality bottle can be had for around five dollars in local supermarkets. That may still sound like a lot of money for vinegar, but in terms of flavor, it's a bargain. Just a little bit lends an elegant, complex sweet-and-sour taste to a wide variety of foods, without adding a drop of fat.

Balsamic vinegar is still aged in wooden casks in Italy, but thanks to technological improvements, only about four years are needed for a good result. It's aged with skins from grapes used to make red wine, which gives it its winelike sweetness (although the vinegar is alcohol-free).

Buying Tips

The longer it's aged, the more mellow it becomes, so check labels.

Serving Ideas

- Sprinkle on salad; an aged balsamic is mellow enough to stand on its own as a salad dressing.
- You-have-to-try-it-to-believe-it department: Pour over fresh strawberries or a melon-ball salad. The fruit's sweetness, combined with the wine flavor and vinegary tang, create an incredible eating experience.
- Marinate vegetables or chicken in a combo of balsamic vinegar, a little olive oil, garlic and basil. It's a great marinade for mushrooms, too.
- When replacing regular vinegar with balsamic, you can use a lot less of the balsamic, it's so flavorful.

Broccoflower

Look! Over in the produce section! Is it a broccoli? Is it a cauliflower? No, it's Broccoflower (also called "Green Cauliflower" and other names), the neon-green hybrid from California that combines the best of both worlds. It's sweet and mild, without the "cabbagey" flavor that turns some people off from cauliflower. It's also softer than broccoli, which means it's easier to chew.

The newfangled crucifer is also a nutritional wonder. Each serving contains hefty vitamin C levels (as much as 125 percent of the RDA, which puts it on a par with broccoli), generous amounts of folic acid (42 percent of the RDA) and more heart-helping beta-carotene than broccoli or cauliflower, according to university research sponsored by the leading grower. As a cruciferous vegetable, it includes other compounds, most notably indoles, that researchers believe may help prevent some kinds of cancer.

Once you've identified Broccoflower, you'll find that

it's easy to recognize. It has a glorious lime coloring, and the buds grow in a symmetrical spiral pattern. (Kids will be fascinated.)

Buying Tips

The florets don't tell you if the head is fresh or not— they hold their color nearly eternally. Broccoflower is past its prime if the jacket leaves are wilted, yellow or limp.

Serving Ideas

• Serve it raw, with a yogurt dip. With its unusual color and pattern, it makes a festive, easy-to-crunch appetizer.
• Add to soups and salads, stir-fries, steamed combinations, casseroles and more.
• Steam and sprinkle with herbs and a grating of Parmesan cheese.

Broccoli Rabe

With a few small broccoli-like florets surrounded by masses of dark green leaves, this green looks innocent enough. But it packs quite a bite with its bitter pungency and just a hint of sweetness.

But don't turn down broccoli rabe on nutritional grounds. This Italian favorite is rich in beta-carotene and vitamin C, with just 27 calories per ½-cup serving.

Buying Tips

Look for firm, small stalks, dark green leaves and green buds.

Serving Ideas

• The classic Italian preparation involves sautéing in oil and garlic. You can get a nearly identical effect with less fat by using an olive-oil pan spray and garlic. After sautéing, add a little water or broth, put a lid on it and let it steam a few more minutes.

Carambola

Cultivated since ancient times in Asia and India, carambola (commonly called star fruit) is just beginning to achieve well-deserved fame in U.S. supermarkets. About the size of a large avocado, the fruit is a glossy yellow oval, with four to six ridges that run lengthwise. Slice crosswise, and—voilà!—golden-yellow stars.

But star fruit is more than just a pretty face. Crunch into it and your reward is a generous spray of aromatic, mildly citruslike juice, which can be very sweet or lightly tart, depending on the individual fruit.

It's a nutritional star, too. With almost no fat, star fruit is a significant source of potassium (207 milligrams per fruit) and vitamin C (27 milligrams per fruit, which is about 45 percent of the RDA). A single fruit contains only about 40 calories.

Buying Tips

Select firm, shiny-skinned fruit. Browning just along the ribbed edges is okay; that's a sign the fruit is ripe. Although it can be eaten when greenish, for full flavor wait for an overall golden-yellow color.

Serving Ideas

• To eat out of hand, just rinse and slice—the skin needn't be peeled.

• Try star fruit in a winter fruit cup, along with oranges, grapefruit and ugli-fruit sections.

• Add slices to spinach salad.

• Chop star fruit into chunks and mix with lime juice and other seasonings for a grilled fish sauce.

• It dresses up a stir-fry, too; add it at the very end and cook only long enough for the fruit to be heated through. (Stir gently, if at all, so the stars won't break.)

• Freeze unused slices for snacks or future fruit salads.

Celery Root

Celery root, or celeriac, looks like what it is, a root, and a knobby, misshapen, often muddy one at that. That's probably why so many shoppers walk on by. But next time you see this funny brown ball, stop and take a whiff. The delicate, celery-like aroma declares that there's more here than meets the eye.

Celeriac comes from a celery-like plant, of which only the root is edible. Raw, it has a light celery flavor, but when cooked, it adds a lot of depth and mellowness to soups and stews. Pretty good for a veggie that contains almost no fat and about 30 calories per ½ cup and is rich in potassium.

Buying Tips

Choose small to medium roots that are as smooth as possible, for easiest peeling.

Serving Ideas

● Julienne, grate or shred for salads. In the French countryside, a celery-root appetizer is traditional fare, julienned and served alongside slices of beets, carrots and tomatoes with a vinaigrette.

● Boil and mash it with potatoes, for an interesting variation on an old favorite.

● Add it to vegetable soups and stews, along with other root vegetables. While it adds deep flavor, it doesn't overwhelm the other flavors.

● Steam or stir-fry chunks of it and serve with horseradish for a zesty, flavorful side dish or appetizer. Keep cooking time brief—10 to 15 minutes are all that's needed once it's peeled and sliced.

Corn and Wheat Tortillas

If the word *tortilla* has always meant "deep fried" to you, it's time to reconsider. The fresh corn and wheat tortillas that are starting to fly off supermarket shelves can be a boon to tasty, low-fat eating.

It's true that in a long list of Mexican dishes, from enchiladas to tostadas, the tortillas are fried in oil. But they can also be microwaved, toasted or baked with little or no fat added, to make your own healthy versions of Mexican— or Italian, or American—favorites. A corn tortilla contains about 1 gram of fat, along with trace minerals. A flour tortilla may contain between 2 and 3 grams of fat, with trace minerals.

Buying Tips

Freshly made tortillas are very conspicuous in supermarkets that serve a Latino population; they can fill many unrefrigerated shelves. In other supermarkets, they're not so easy to find; search refrigerated cases, like the dairy case and even the meat case.

Always check the ingredients list first before buying. Some flour tortillas contain added shortening or oil.

Serving Ideas

• Flour tortillas are soft and easily rolled for sandwiches. Corn tortillas, with their bonus corn flavor, have a harder texture and don't roll quite as easily, but they're ideal for open-faced sandwiches.

• Tortillas can be warmed and softened on a paper towel in the microwave in a few seconds. Or place tortillas in a nonstick pan and toast—no oil needed. Some people toast their corn tortillas over an open gas flame (proceed with caution!). Then, add your favorite ingredients—from peanut butter and jelly to stir-fried vegetables—and enjoy!

• For fast, low-fat nacho chips: Make several cuts in corn tortillas from five or six points on the perimeter to about an

inch from the center. Heat oven to 350°F. Place corn tortillas on oven rack and bake for five to seven minutes, checking frequently to avoid burning. Remove, break apart and
serve with chunky salsa!

● Throw a make-it-yourself fajita dinner. Marinate chicken,
turkey or beef strips in lime juice, garlic and red chilies for
an hour. Broil or sauté the meat. Set the plate of cooked
meat on the table, along with tortillas, small bowls of salsa,
shredded lettuce, yogurt, sprouts, cooked beans, cooked
potatoes, brown rice, chopped onions, chopped cilantro
and guacamole. Everyone rolls their own dinner!

● Try a "Mexican pizza": Top a corn tortilla with tomato
slices or tomato sauce, chopped onions, green peppers,
jalapeños and grated low-fat cheese.

● Scrambled egg whites or egg substitutes are delicious
rolled in a tortilla. Scramble with onions and green or red
peppers and add a dash of hot sauce, if you dare.

● Make broccoli quesadillas: Sauté broccoli, tomatoes, jalapeño peppers and scallions. Place on flour tortillas; roll
up and cook in a no-stick pan with a little olive-oil spray.

Cultivated Exotic Mushrooms

Question: What's as satisfying to chew as meat,
loaded with subtle and amazing flavors, and contains very
little fat or calories? Answer: the new breed of exotic mushrooms.

Exotic mushrooms are easier to find and less expensive than ever before, since there's been a cultivation boom
in the United States. The mushrooms are available both
fresh and dried, and there are good reasons to keep both
kinds on hand.

Among our favorite fresh varieties: Shiitake mushrooms (pronounced *shee-ee-TOCK-ee*). These parasol-
shaped brownish-black mushrooms have a light garlic-
pine aroma. They also offer the meatiest texture and flavor,
along with trace amounts of minerals and B vitamins.

And some other marvelous mushrooms. Oyster mushrooms have luscious, large, shell-shaped caps and a light seafood flavor when cooked. Enoki are delicate, creamy-white mushrooms, with tiny caps and long stems—the Japanese float them in broth. Chantarelles are as enchanting as their name. Shaped like a trumpet flower, they can range in color from orange to black, with a flavor that can be nutty, cinnamon-like or fruity like an apricot. And the list of mushrooms goes on and on.

Dried mushrooms have two important virtues: They keep for a long time in a cool, dry place; and they can produce a nearly instant, flavorful, no-fat broth, much like beef stock. Among the popular dried varieties available in supermarkets: shiitake, porcini, oyster, wood ear, cepe, chantarelle and the highly prized (and priced to match) morel. They can be reconstituted and then prepared like fresh mushrooms.

Buying Tips

Choose fresh varieties that show no sign of deterioration. They should be firm and plump to the touch. When you get them home, store unwashed in a brown paper bag or on a plate covered with damp paper towels or cheesecloth in the refrigerator.

Dried mushrooms, often found in small packages in the produce department, can be kept indefinitely at room temperature in a dry place.

Serving Ideas

● To reconstitute dried mushrooms, place in warm or boiled water for 20 minutes. Reserve the liquid, filtered through cheesecloth or a coffee filter, to use as a stock.
● Slice mushrooms for salads. Or marinate them in balsamic vinegar and then add to salads.
● Mushrooms are a natural "meat extender." Stir-fry shiitake with vegetables and a little chicken, turkey or meat for a low-fat entrée.

• Sautéed exotic mushrooms are an impressive appetizer. Use a no-stick spray, or cook them in a small amount of broth from reconstituted dried mushrooms. Sauté with sliced, roasted, skinned red peppers for a pleasant tang.

• Make a glaze for meats, using defatted chicken broth to rehydrate dried mushrooms. Reduce to a syrupy consistency in a saucepan.

• Add dried mushrooms when you begin cooking a rice pilaf; they add flavor and texture—and serve as a garnish! (Include other seasonings, like sautéed leeks or thyme leaves.) By the time the pilaf is cooked, the mushrooms will be fully reconstituted.

• Splurge and try morels; they have an earthy flavor reminiscent of hazelnuts and a spongelike texture that will enslave your tongue. Sauté and serve alone, or use to make sauces for meat or fish.

Flash-Frozen Fish

Imagine having fresh, tender, top-quality fillets of fish any time you want them, without living next to an ocean. It's possible, thanks to new freezing technology by which fresh-caught fish are quick-frozen, shrink-wrapped and sent to supermarket freezer cases.

The hitch: This technology is expensive, so only a few companies do it, and the prices reflect that—comparable to prices for good-quality cuts of meat.

But converts say the cost is well worth it. *Prevention* editors broiled up high-tech mahimahi and swordfish steaks and found it nearly impossible to believe that they'd been frozen. The flesh was so moist and fresh that we could have been eating in a pier-side restaurant.

That's no surprise, say the manufacturers. The fish is frozen within hours of being caught and stays that way until you're ready to prepare it. You can't get much fresher than that, unless you're on board a fishing boat.

What's more, since the technology is expensive, the

◆

companies use the best cuts of fish only, so that customers are willing to pay extra. That means you can be more certain of a top-quality fish.

Buying Tips

Vacuum-sealed frozen fish is distinctive: A thick layer of transparent plastic clings so tightly to the fillet that the wrapping is virtually invisible. (One astonished cashier tried to scratch our fillet to determine whether it really was wrapped!) Because of the cost, distribution is limited: Find it in the freezer case of upscale supermarkets.

Serving Ideas

• Follow package directions for defrosting. You can do anything with this fish that you'd do with fresh: broil, bake, grill, poach, barbecue, steam or microwave.

Jicama

Tired of plain old carrot and celery crudités? Add jicama (pronounced *HEE-keh-mah*) to the pack. This brown, round, rough-skinned root features a snowy-white interior with a very mild and juicy-sweet apple flavor.

Jicama provides a lot of crunch for a few calories: A ½-cup serving contains less than 25 calories. It has 12 milligrams of vitamin C—about 20 percent of the RDA—and small amounts of minerals and B vitamins.

Buying Tips

Jicamas can range from apple to cantaloupe size. Select ones with thin skins, because thick-skinned jicama can be fibrous and starchy. Always peel the skin before eating or cooking.

Serving Ideas

• For appealing appetizers, julienne or cut into ¼-inch-thick slices. (For parties, cut the slices into various shapes with a cookie cutter.) It's ideal with a yogurt dip; the tangy sourness of the yogurt contrasts nicely with a jicama's sweetness.

● For a Latin-style appetizer, peel and slice jicama into ¼-inch slices; sprinkle with chopped red chilies, garnish with a few sprigs of fresh cilantro and chill for two hours. Serve with fresh lime slices for guests to squeeze on top.

● Julienned, shredded or grated, raw jicama adds flavor and visual appeal to fruit and vegetable salads.

● Stir-fry or steam it briefly—it stands in for water chest-nuts, because it stays crisp when cooked.

New Turkey Cuts

Once upon a time, a fresh turkey dinner required a cook to spend a half-day toiling by a hot oven. But with the appearance of new skinless and boneless turkey thighs, cutlets and tenderloins, a hearty, healthy, family turkey din-ner can appear in a few minutes.

Turkey has a distinctively rich, robust flavor that lends a festive feeling even to workday meals. Better yet, it's very low in fat—lower even than chicken. Turkey tenderloins and cutlets—both breast meat—are less than 5 percent fat; skinless turkey thighs are 20 percent fat, roughly the same as chicken breast.

Buying Tips

Look in the refrigerated meat case for the following cuts:

● Turkey cutlets, which are slices off the breast about ½-inch thick.

● Turkey tenderloins (also called fillets), which are thicker strips of breast meat that include the entire muscle from the inside center of the breast.

● Thigh steaks (dark meat from the turkey thigh) and drumstick steaks.

Some of these cuts are packaged by national manufacturers; others are prepared by the supermarket. Check expiration dates to assure freshness.

Serving Ideas
• An easy way to prepare turkey cutlets: Spray a no-stick pan with cooking spray, sprinkle cutlets with your choice of seasonings—sage, thyme or rosemary, or an Italian or Cajun spice blend—and cook two to three minutes on each side. During the last minute of cooking time, add ⅓ cup of liquid, such as broth or fruit juice.
• Cut turkey cutlets into strips, cook and chill for salads.
• Turkey breast tenderloins can be cut crosswise into round or oval-shaped medallions. Or serve them whole, baked or stuffed, for company.
• Thin-slice turkey for stir-fry; cube it for kabobs and casseroles.
• Make a quick, substantial rice-and-bean turkey stew: In a cast-iron pot, sauté chopped onions in a small amount of olive oil; add turkey tenderloins and brown. Add two cups of defatted chicken broth, a cup of quick ten-minute brown rice and a can of pinto beans. Season with a pinch of cumin and oregano. Bring to a boil, reduce heat to simmer, and cover. Ready in ten minutes.

Quince
Close your eyes and imagine the best baked apple that you possibly can. Sink your teeth into chunks that are sweet yet tart, firm yet pliant, moist and juicy all at once.

It's rare to get a baked apple that good. But there's one way that's virtually guaranteed: Instead of an apple, bake a quince.

Raw, quince is so sour and dry as to be virtually inedible. But cooking transforms it into food for the angels.

Healthy angels, that is. Quince is fat-free, offers 14 milligrams of vitamin C per fruit (about 23 percent of the RDA) and small amounts of minerals and B vitamins.

Buying Tips

Quinces are usually found near the apples. Each looks like a large bumpy green or yellow apple, with the stem end protruding slightly. The fruit should be hard; cooking softens it.

Serving Ideas

- Slice and simmer in sauces.
- Bake like an apple with cinnamon and raisins.
- Cook with chicken, duck or ham.
- It's a favorite in fruit tarts since it holds its shape, not dissolving as easily as apples.
- Add some quince to a fruit compote—along with apples, pears, kumquats, bananas—and zap for 12 minutes in the microwave.

Sweet Winter Squash

Next time you see UFOs hovering around the winter squash section of your supermarket, don't call Geraldo; take one home. True, these Unidentified Furrowed Objects have bumpy skin that's green, blue, red or yellow. But on the inside they offer a familiar treasure of beta-carotene, with few calories, in a delicious form. More delicious than ever, in fact.

New varieties are appearing constantly in the supermarket, and among them are some that are just outstanding in flavor and texture.

One of our new favorites: delicata squash, shaped like a large zucchini with red, white, yellow and green stripes on the outside. The larger-sized delicata, over seven inches or so, are excellent, but the smaller ones are ambrosia: When baked, they're so sweet and creamy that they could stand as a dessert pudding, with no brown sugar added. (And the skin on the small ones is edible.)

Another favorite: Sweet dumpling squash is shaped like a flat-bottomed acorn squash, and its skin also features a sunset palette of yellows, oranges, reds and greens. It tastes like sweet toasted almonds, with a firm, rich flesh that's practically addictive.

Buying Tips

Don't be afraid to experiment. Each squash variety offers different flavors and degrees of sweetness. Sweet newcomers include sweet dumpling, delicata, kabocha (Japanese squash) and sweet Chinese.

Avoid squash with obvious bruises or soft spots. They should feel heavy for their size. Both delicata and sweet dumpling squash are ready for eating when their white stripes have turned completely yellow.

Serving Ideas

● Squash can be grilled. Slice thick and marinate with soy sauce and a little rice-wine vinegar and sesame oil. Precook for a few minutes in the oven or microwave, and finish on the grill.
● Sauté chunks of squash with defatted chicken broth, toss with onions (cooked in broth over low heat until they soften), then add caraway seeds toasted in a dry pan, and nutmeg.
● Top warm, sweet varieties with low-fat frozen yogurt or ice cream.

How Healthy Is Your Diet? Take This Test

We all know that eating a diet low in cholesterol and saturated fat lowers blood levels of cholesterol and reduces our risk of heart disease. But knowing that doesn't necessarily make it easy to choose what to eat.

So the husband-and-wife team of William Connor, M.D., and Sonja Connor, M.S., R.D., created the Cholesterol–Saturated Fat Index (CSI), a system that makes it simple for us to pick the foods that are least likely to raise cholesterol. With their colleagues at the Oregon Health Sciences Center in Portland, they assigned one number, the CSI, to hundreds of foods—basics as well as brand-name prepared foods. The lower the CSI, the better the food is for you. The CSI rates the heart-healthiness of each food. It also eliminates the confusion surrounding things like shrimp (CSI 9), which is high in cholesterol but low in saturated fat, and tropical vegetable oils like palm (CSI 54) and coconut (CSI 95) oils, that have no cholesterol but lots of saturated fat.

But the Connors have gone far beyond just assigning numbers to foods. They studied the eating habits of 233 average American families for several years and worked out a way to calculate the CSI of whole diets, too.

How high is your daily CSI? And how high *should* it be if you want to improve your rating under the CSI system? To answer both questions, simply take the quiz on these pages, which is from the Connors' book, *The New American Diet System.* Once you know your number, you can make changes in the way you eat to get it down to a healthier level.

Directions

Under each food category listed below, you will find a number of questions, and for each question there are a number of possible answers or choices. Circle the numbers to the left of the choices that best describe your eating habits during the past month. Put that number in the blank space labeled "score" after each question. If you circle more than one choice for a single question, put the lowest score circled in the blank. For example, if you circle number 1, number 2 and number 3 under question 5 in the Meat, Fish and Poultry portion of the quiz, your score is 1, which is the score you should enter for question 5. Some questions are worded in such a way that it is likely you will have only one answer; that's the case with question 4 under the Meat, Fish and Poultry category, for example.

When you have computed the score for each question in a category (such as Meat, Fish and Poultry), add all of those scores together to arrive at your total score for each category. Then see "Computing Your Daily CSI Score" (page 85) and "What Do Your Quiz Scores Mean?" (page 87) to find out what to do with those scores.

Meat, Fish and Poultry

For each question, circle as many numbers as apply. Your score for each question is the lowest number circled.

1. Which type of ground beef do you usually eat?
1 Regular hamburger (30% fat)
2 Lean ground beef (25% fat)
3 Extra lean/ground chuck (20% fat)
4 Super lean/ground round (15% fat)
5 Ground sirloin (10% fat) or eat no ground beef
SCORE _____

2. Which best describes your typical lunch?
1 Cheeseburger, typical cheeses, egg dishes (egg salad, quiche, etc.)
2 Sandwiches (lunch meat, hot dog, hamburger, fried fish, etc.) or entrée of meat or chicken (plain or fried)
3 Tuna sandwich, fish entrée (not fried), entrée with small bits of chicken or meat in a soup or casserole
4 Peanut butter sandwich
5 Salad, yogurt, cottage cheese, vegetarian dishes (without high-fat cheeses or egg yolk)
SCORE _____

3. Circle all of the choices that characterize the entrées (main courses) at your main meals

1 Cheese (cheddar, Jack, etc.), eggs, liver, heart or brains once a week or more

2 Beef, lamb, pork, or ham once a week or more

3 Very lean red meat (top round or flank steak), veal, venison or elk once a week or more

4 Chicken, turkey, rabbit, crab, lobster or shrimp twice a week or more

5 Fish, scallops, oysters, clams or meatless dishes containing no egg yolk or high-fat cheese twice a week or more

SCORE _____

4. Estimate the number of ounces of meat, cheese, fish and poultry you eat in a typical day. Include all meals and snacks. To guide you in your estimate: 4 strips of bacon = 1 ounce; 1 small burger patty = 3 to 4 ounces; meat in most sandwiches = 2 to 3 ounces; 1 slice of cheese = 1 ounce; 1 chicken thigh = 2 to 3 ounces; ½ chicken breast = 3 ounces; 1 average T-bone steak = 8 ounces; 1-inch cube of cheese = 1 ounce.

1 11 or more ounces a day

2 9 to 10 ounces a day

3 6 to 8 ounces a day

4 4 to 5 ounces a day

5 Not more than 1 ounce of cheese, 3 ounces of red meat, poultry, shrimp, crab, lobster or not more than 6 ounces of fish, clams, oysters, scallops a day

SCORE _____

5. Which of these have you eaten in the past month?

1 Bacon, sausage, bologna and other lunch meats, pepperoni, beef or pork weiners

2 Canadian bacon, turkey wieners

3 Turkey ham and other poultry lunch meats

4 Soy products (breakfast links)
5 None
SCORE _____

TOTAL SCORE _____ (Add the scores from the previous five questions.)

Dairy Products and Eggs

For each question, circle as many numbers as apply. Your score for each question is the lowest number circled.

1. Which kinds of milk do you use for drinking or cooking?
1 Whole milk
2 2% milk
4 1% milk, buttermilk
5 Skim milk, nonfat dry milk or none
SCORE _____

2. Which toppings do you use at least once a month?
1 Sour cream (real or imitation) or whipped cream
3 Nondairy topping (Cool Whip or Dream Whip)
4 Regular cottage cheese, whole-milk yogurt
5 Low-fat cottage cheese, low-fat or nonfat yogurt or none
SCORE _____

3. Which frozen desserts do you eat at least once a month?
1 Ice cream
2 Ice milk, most soft ice cream, Tofutti, frozen yogurt (cream added)
4 Sherbet, low-fat frozen yogurt, Lite Lite Tofutti
5 Sorbets, ices, nonfat frozen yogurt, Popsicles or none
SCORE _____

4. Which kinds of cheese do you use for snacks or sandwiches?

1 Cheddar, Swiss, Jack, Brie, feta, American, cream cheese, regular cheese slices or cheese spreads

2 Part-skim mozzarella, Lappi, light cream cheese or Neufchâtel, part-skim cheddar (Kraft Light, Green River, Olympia's Low Fat or Heidi Ann Low-Fat Ched-Style Cheese)

4 Low-cholesterol "filled" cheese (Scandic Mini Chol [Swedish low cholesterol] or Hickory Farms Lyte)

5 Very-low-fat processed cheese (Dorman's Light, Reduced Calories Laughing Cow, Weight Watchers or the Lite-Line series of cheeses) or none

SCORE _____

5. Which kinds of cheese do you use in cooking (casseroles, vegetables, etc.)?

1 Cheddar, Swiss, Jack, Brie, feta, American, cream cheese, processed cheese (Note: Used in most restaurants)

3 Part-skim mozzarella, Lappi, light cream cheese, part-skim cheddar (Green River, Olympia's Low Fat, Kraft Light, or Heidi Ann Low-Fat Ched-Style Cheese)

4 Low-cholesterol "filled" cheese (Scandic Mini Chol [Swedish low cholesterol] or Hickory Farms Lyte)

5 Very-low-fat processed cheese (Dorman's Light, Reduced Calories Laughing Cow, Weight Watchers or the Lite-Line series of cheeses) or none

SCORE _____

6. Check the type and number of "visible" eggs you eat.

1 6 or more whole eggs a week

2 3 to 5 whole eggs a week

3 1 to 2 whole eggs a week

4   1 whole egg a month

5   Egg white, egg substitute such as Egg Beaters, Scramblers, Second Nature or none
SCORE _____

7.   Check the type of eggs usually used in food prepared at home or bought in grocery stores (baked goods, such as cakes and cookies, potato and pasta salads, pancakes, etc.)

1   Whole eggs or mixes containing whole eggs (complete pancake mix, slice-and-bake cookies, etc.)

3   Combination of egg white, egg substitute and whole egg

5   Egg white, egg substitute or none
SCORE _____

TOTAL SCORE _____ (Add the scores from the previous seven questions.)

Fats and Oils

For each question, circle as many numbers as apply. Your score for each question is the lowest number circled.

1.   Which kinds of fats are used to cook your food (vegetables, meats, etc.)?

1   Butter, shortening (all brands except Crisco or Food Club) or lard, bacon grease, chicken fat or eat in restaurants at least four times a week

3   Soft shortening (Crisco or Food Club) or inexpensive stick margarine

4   Tub or soft-stick margarine, vegetable oil

5   None or use no-stick pan or spray
SCORE _____

2.   Which best describes your daily use of these "visible" fats?

Typical amounts used   *Your use in one day*

- 2 teaspoons margarine, butter on toast (each slice):   ____
- 6 teaspoons mayonnaise on sandwiches (amount/sandwich):   ____
- 6 teaspoons peanut butter on sandwiches (amount/sandwich):   ____
- 2 teaspoons margarine, butter on sandwiches (amount/sandwich):
- 12 teaspoons regular salad dressings on salads: ____
- 3 to 6 teaspoons margarine, butter on potatoes: ____
- 3 teaspoons margarine, butter on vegetables: ____

Total: ____ teaspoons

1 10 teaspoons or more
2 8 to 9 teaspoons
3 6 to 7 teaspoons
4 4 to 5 teaspoons
5 3 teaspoons or less
SCORE _____

3. How often do you eat potato chips, corn or tortilla chips, fried chicken, fish sticks, French fries, doughnuts, other fried foods, croissants or Danish pastries?

1 Two or more times a day
2 Once a day
3 Two to four times a week
4 Once a week
5 Less than twice a month
SCORE _____

4. Which best describes the amount of margarine, peanut butter, mayonnaise or cream cheese that you put on breads, muffins, bagels, etc.?

1 Average (1 teaspoon or more per serving)
2 Lightly spread (can see through it)

    4 "Scrape" (can barely see it)
    5 None
SCORE _____

    5. Which kind of salad dressings do you use?
    1 Real mayonnaise
    2 Miracle Whip, ranch, French, Roquefort, blue cheese and vinegar and oil dressings
    3 Light mayonnaise, Miracle Whip Light, Thousand Island dressing
    4 Russian and Italian dressings, ranch salad dressing made with buttermilk and light mayonnaise or Miracle Whip Light
    5 Low-calorie dressing, vinegar, lemon juice, ranch dressing made with buttermilk and nonfat or low-fat yogurt or use lemon or no salad dressing
    SCORE _____

    TOTAL SCORE _____ (Add the scores from the previous five questions.)

Sweets and Snacks
    For each question, circle as many numbers as apply. Your score for each question is the lowest number circled.

    1. How often do you eat dessert or baked goods (sweet rolls, doughnuts, cookies, cakes, etc.)?
    1 Three or more times a day
    2 Two times a day
    3 Once a day
    4 Four to six times a week
    5 Three or four times a week or less
    SCORE _____

    2. Which of the following are you most likely to select as a dessert choice?

1   Croissants, pies, cheesecake, carrot cake
2   Regular cakes, cupcakes, cookies
4   Low-fat muffins, desserts from low-fat cookbooks or none
5   Fruits, low-fat cookies (fig bars, vanilla wafers, graham crackers and gingersnaps), angel food cake
SCORE _____

3. Which snack items are you most likely to eat in an average month?
1   Chocolate
2   Potato chips, corn or tortilla chips, nuts, party/snack crackers, doughnuts, french fries, peanut butter, cookies
4   Lightly "buttered" popcorn (1 teaspoon margarine for three cups), pretzels, low-fat crackers (soda, graham), "homebaked" corn chips, low-fat cookies (gingersnaps, fig bars)
5   Fruit, vegetables, very low-fat snacks or none
SCORE _____

TOTAL SCORE _____ (Add the scores from the previous three questions.)

Computing Your Daily CSI Score

First add up all your scores from the different parts of the test to get a "combined" score.

Then, if you're a woman or are doing this for a child, read Part 2, on page 86. It will tell you how to translate your combined score into a daily CSI number.

If you're a teenager or a man, see Part 3 for instructions on turning your combined score into a daily CSI.

Part 1: Calculating Your Combined Score
Add your scores from all four parts of the quiz.

Meat, Fish and Poultry   ____
Dairy Products and Eggs   ____
Fats and Oils   ____
Sweets and Snacks   ____
COMBINED SCORE   ____

Part 2: For Women and Children
Here are the steps for turning your combined score into a daily CSI:

• If your combined score is 57 or less, your daily CSI is 51. Sorry. You're eating a typical American diet.
• If your combined score is 58 to 70, your daily CSI is 37. You're in Phase One. Congratulations; you're on your way.
• If your combined score is 71 to 86, your daily CSI is 28, and you're in Phase Two.
• If your combined score is 87 or more, your daily CSI is 16. Phase Three: You've made it to the mountaintop.

Part 3: For Men and Teenagers
Here are the steps for turning your combined score into a daily CSI:

• If your combined score is 55 or less, your daily CSI is 69. Sorry. You're eating a typical American diet.
• If your combined score is 56 to 68, your daily CSI is 49. You're in Phase One. Congratulations; you're on your way.
• If your combined score is 69 to 84, your daily CSI is 36, and you're in Phase Two.
• If your combined score is 87 or more, your daily CSI is 16. Phase Three: You've made it to the mountaintop.

What Do Your Quiz Scores Mean?

You've taken the test. You've computed your score. Now it's time to find out what those scores mean.

If you're a woman and your daily CSI is 51, or if you're a man and your daily CSI is 69, then you will want to start modifying your diet considerably, but gradually.

If, on the other hand, your combined score places you into the Phase One CSI category, you're already on your way to a healthier diet. If your combined score places you in Phase Two, you're not only on your way, you're doing very well indeed. Keep up the good work. And if you're in Phase Three, you're a nutritional champion.

You'll want to take this quiz over again from time to time as you gradually make lower CSI food choices and thus adapt to a lower-fat, lower-cholesterol style of eating. Remember, as your CSI goes down, so does your risk of heart disease, stroke, obesity and some cancers, such as breast and colon cancers.

Moving from One Phase to Another

When you move from a typical American diet to achieve a Phase One CSI, going from 51 to 37 for women or from 69 to 49 for men, say the Connors, "You will have reduced your cholesterol intake, on average, from 400 to 500 milligrams per day to 300 to 350 milligrams. Fat intake will be reduced from 40 percent of calories to 30 percent (with saturated fat going from 14 percent to 10 percent). On average, these changes will result in up to a 6 percent reduction in your blood cholesterol level and a 12 percent reduction in the risk of coronary heart disease.

"When you achieve a Phase Two CSI of 28 [women] or 36 [men]," they continue, "your cholesterol intake will average about 200 milligrams daily, and the fat content of your diet will be only 25 percent of calories (with just 8 percent of calories in the form of saturated fat). These changes can reduce your blood cholesterol level by up to 13 percent and your risk of coronary heart disease by up to 26 percent."

And if you achieve a Phase Three CSI of 16 for women or 23 for men, they say, "your diet will consist of 20 percent fat (only 5 percent of the calories will be saturated fat), and your cholesterol level will be reduced up to 20 percent, and your risk of coronary heart disease will be reduced by up to 40 percent!"

Healthy Lunches Are in the Bag

These days lots of people are packing lunch to take to school or work, because it's hard to rely on restaurants and cafeterias for low-fat cuisine. It's also a lot less expensive to bag lunch than to ring up that lunch bill five days a week. If you're thinking about cutting fat and want to start packing lunch more often, try these tips for making healthy, nutritious portable lunches.

These days a sandwich builder can choose from low-fat cheeses and no-added-sugar peanut butters and fruit spreads. Even cold cuts have come in from the cold. There are many you can choose from that have under 1 gram of fat per ounce. That means even a fairly substantial sandwich, with two ounces or so of meat in it, weighs in with only 2 grams of fat.

So a sandwich made with two slices of Oscar Mayer Oven-Roasted Chicken Breast, for example, on two pieces of whole wheat bread with lettuce and ½ tablespoon of nonfat mayo has only 3.4 grams of fat and gets only 15 percent of its calories from fat. Even if you made a more hefty version of the same sandwich with three or four slices of the chicken breast, it would have only 17 percent of its calories from fat.

Leaner, But Still Salty

Unfortunately, while meat packers have cut the fat, they haven't done nearly as well at reducing the sodium in their products. Most of these meats tend to have fairly high amounts of sodium, both because it is a preservative and because it enhances the admittedly rather bland flavors of turkey and chicken. (But we think one of the tastiest brands is Weaver's, which has the least sodium of all.)

Kids don't need more than 300 to 500 milligrams of sodium per day, depending on their age. But although there is no known link between childhood salt intake and adult high blood pressure, it's prudent for everyone to limit salt intake. So you may want to select the lower-sodium brands.

The Nitrate Issue

Nitrates are another food additive that seem almost impossible to avoid in lunch meats. They are added to prevent spoilage and retain the appetizing color of the meat.

The whole issue of whether or not nitrosamines (the substances that nitrates are changed into in our bodies) are a major risk factor for some types of cancer is still unanswered. Still, the American Cancer Society recommends limiting your intake of nitrate-cured meats, unless they have vitamin C compounds added. The vitamin C is believed to keep nitrates from turning into cancer-causing chemicals. Look for the term "ascorbic acid," "sodium ascorbate" or "sodium erythrobate" on the label.

Cold Cuts That Make the Grade

All the lunch meats listed here have 1 gram of fat—or less—in one ounce, so they're very good selections for sandwich meat. We ranked these products according to the fat they contain, not the percentage of calories from fat.

If you're salt-sensitive (according to your doctor), then you should choose a brand that packs less than 250 milligrams of sodium per ounce.

Meat	Slices per 1 oz.	Calories	Fat (g)	Calories from Fat (%)	Nitrate (mg)
Hillshire Farm Deli-Select Oven-Roast Turkey Breast	3.0	30	0.3	9	300
Oscar Mayer Smoked Turkey Breast	1.4	28	0.3	10	308
Louis Rich Deli-Thin Smoked Turkey Breast	2.5	25	0.3	11	275
Hillshire Farm Deli-Select Smoked Turkey Breast	3.0	30	0.4	12	300
Weaver Turkey Breast	1.0	29	0.4	12	197
Oscar Mayer Thin-Sliced Turkey Roast	2.4	36	0.5	13	360
Mr. Turkey Smoked Turkey Breast	1.0	33	0.5	14	332
Hillshire Farm Deli-Select Pastrami	3.0	30	0.5	15	300
Hillshire Farm Deli-Select Smoked Beef	3.0	30	0.5	15	270
Oscar Mayer Corned Beef	1.7	26	0.5	17	349
Oscar Mayer Pastrami	1.7	26	0.5	17	365
Oscar Mayer Thin-Sliced Smoked Turkey	2.4	24	0.5	19	288
Oscar Mayer Baked Ham	1.4	28	0.7	23	336

Meat	Slices per 1 oz.	Calories	Fat (g)	Calories from Fat (%)	Nitrate (mg)
Oscar Mayer Oven-Roasted Turkey Breast	1.4	28	0.7	23	252
Oscar Mayer Honey Ham	1.4	35	0.8	21	371
Mr. Turkey Chicken Breast	1.0	33	0.9	25	190
Hillshire Farm Deli-Select Cajun Ham	3.0	30	0.9	27	360
Mr. Turkey Turkey Pastrami	1.0	28	0.9	29	383
Butterball Turkey Ham	1.0	35	1.0	26	390
Louis Rich Honey-Cured Turkey Ham	1.4	34	1.0	26	290
Louis Rich Honey-Roast Turkey Breast	1.0	35	1.0	26	315
Louis Rich Oven-Roasted White Chicken	1.0	35	1.0	26	285
Oscar Mayer Boiled Ham	1.4	35	1.0	26	385
Butterball Smoked Turkey Breast	1.0	30	1.0	30	230
Eckrich Lite Oven-Roasted Turkey Breast	1.0	30	1.0	30	210
Eckrich Lite Smoked Chicken Breast	1.0	30	1.0	30	210
Emmber Lean 'n' Tender Italian Beef	1.0	30	1.0	30	270
Emmber Lean 'n' Tender Pork Roast	1.0	30	1.0	30	230
Louis Rich Deluxe Oven-Roasted Chicken Breast	1.0	30	1.0	30	330
Russer Lil'Salt Ham	1.0	30	1.0	30	220
Alpine Lace Cooked Ham	1.0	25	1.0	36	220
Alpine Lace Smoked Ham	1.0	25	1.0	36	220
Eckrich Lite Cooked Ham	1.0	25	1.0	36	360
Louis Rich Deli-Thin Turkey Pastrami (round)	2.5	25	1.0	36	313
Oscar Mayer Oven-Roasted Chicken Breast	1.0	25	1.0	36	270

Cold Cuts Too Fatty to Favor

If bologna did have a first name it would be f-a-t-t-y. But the old lunchbox standbys aren't the only cold cuts that have too much fat to be daily fare. As you can see on this table, products made with chicken or turkey aren't automatically low fat. Notice too that although these cold cuts may not be great shakes in the fat department, some of them have terrifically low levels of sodium.

Meat	Slices per 1 oz.	Calories	Fat (g)	Calories from Fat (%)	Nitrate (mg)
Oscar Mayer Hard Salami	3	105	9	77	510
Oscar Mayer Bologna	1	90	8	80	320
Mr. Turkey Turkey Bologna	1	63	6	86	247
Weaver Chicken Bologna	1	68	6	79	284
Butterball Turkey Bologna	1	70	6	77	340
Eckrich Light Bologna	1	70	6	77	250
Oscar Mayer Luncheon Loaf	1	75	6	72	345
Russer Lil'Salt Bologna	1	70	5	64	200
Oscar Mayer Pickle and Pimiento Loaf	1	65	4	55	370
Russer Lil'Salt Old-Fashioned Loaf	1	60	3	45	200

Researched by Diane Drabinsky, R.D.

Read the Label

One cold cut that the manufacturers haven't seen fit to tinker with (or haven't figured out how to defat) is the kid classic, bologna. No matter what it's made from—turkey, chicken or beef—bologna is a nutritional disaster, with as much as eight times more fat than any of the more healthy choices. It's also laced with sodium.

This illustrates another important point about this new generation of poultry-based lunch meats: Just because they're made with chicken or turkey doesn't mean the final products are low in fat. You have to read the labels. Any brand that has more than 1 gram of fat per ounce is not your best choice.

Building a Better Sandwich

Sandwiches are the easiest and most convenient anchor for a brown bag lunch. But it's all too easy to get into a rut and pack the same old thing every day. This year, why not break out of the ordinary—and pack some extra nutrition as well. Use the lists below to expand your lunchtime horizons. Pick one ingredient from each of the first three lists, then add as many extras as you like. And you can round out your lunch with any of the accompaniments in the last list.

Breads

- Whole grain bread: rye, pumpernickel, multigrain, herb
- English muffin
- Bagel
- Pita bread
- Flour tortilla
- Italian roll
- French bread
- WASA crispbread
- Kaiser roll
- Rice cakes
- Popcorn cakes

Condiments

- Reduced-calorie mayonnaise
- Mustard: Dijon, Parisian, hot, honey, coarse
- Low-fat salad dressing: French, Italian, Russian, ranch
- Flavored vinegars: balsamic, tarragon
- Herbal soft cheese
- Horseradish
- Tahini dressing
- Fruit butters

Fillings

- Grilled chicken cutlet
- Bean spread
- Tuna salad
- Chicken salad
- Seafood salad
- Hummus
- Sliced lean meat
- Smoked salmon
- Low-fat peanut butter
- Low-fat sliced cheese

Extras

- Lettuce: escarole, endive, Romaine, leaf, Boston
- Red onion
- Tomato slices
- Avocado slices
- Low-fat cheese, grated
- Cucumber slices
- Spinach
- Sweet pepper rings: green, red, yellow, purple
- Mushrooms, sliced

- Carrot, grated
- Red and green cabbage, grated
- Watercress
- Red beets, grated
- Jicama, grated
- Sesame seeds, toasted
- Sprouts: alfalfa, mung bean, radish

Accompaniments

- Fresh fruit
- Mini rice cakes: plain, teriyaki, honey nut, barbe-cue, nacho, ranch
- Popcorn, air popped
- Pretzels
- Fruit leathers
- Fresh vegetable sticks
- Pasta salad
- Rice salad
- Tossed salad with low-fat dressing
- Soup, hot or cold
- Three-bean salad
- Coleslaw
- Pickled cabbage
- Potato salad
- Carrot-raisin salad
- Marinated vegetables
- Dried fruit: raisins, apples, apricots, figs, etc.
- Graham crackers
- Animal crackers
- Fig bars
- Pickled red beets
- Low-fat pudding: regular, tapioca, rice
- Low-fat and nonfat yogurt: plain, fruited, flavored
- Fruit juice
- Water

- Seltzer
- Fruit juice sparkler
- Mineral water: plain or flavored
- Vegetable juice
- Low-fat milk
- Lemonade
- Iced herbal tea

Making the Grade: A Red-Meat Primer for the Fat Conscious

You still get your iced tea in glass cowboy-boot mugs, but first choice in beef isn't what it used to be at the Big Texan Steak Ranch in Amarillo. Even cattlemen are cutting back these days, according to the waitress.

Big Texan's most often ordered meal is no longer the 42-ounce marathon steak or even the 14-ounce Texas T-bone. Ranchers, oilmen, tourists and truckers passing on I-40 now request the "Wichita Falls" prime, a smaller, 7-ounce serving.

Big Texan's popular slimmed-down portion is still about twice the serving size nutritionists recommend for healthwise dining. But it does signal a growing health trend: Concerned about the effects of cholesterol and saturated fat in our diet, we Americans are trimming our red meat intake.

The (Flip) Side of Beef

For a nation that has long ranked steak right up there with Mom and apple pie, a little conservatism is certainly healthy. But before you cut your meat intake to the bone, consider this:

• In our vast food kingdom, red meat reigns supreme in iron content. Beef contains at least 1½ times more iron than an equivalent serving of chicken or fish. Pork and lamb contain more iron than an equal amount of chicken. And, unlike the iron in vegetables, fruits and grains, the iron in red meat is readily absorbed by the body. What's more, by including a small amount of red meat in a mostly grain-and-vegetable meal, you will actually increase the iron availability from the nonmeat sources.

• Meat helps build strong bones. It contains substantial amounts of copper, manganese and zinc. These three minerals work together with calcium to prevent the brittle-bone condition known as osteoporosis. Beef, in particular, is a veritable banquet for the bones; it's high in copper and manganese. Beef, pork and lamb are all good sources of zinc.

• Red meat is an excellent source of B-complex vitamins and protein.

New Meat-Eating Perspective

Don't take all this as carte blanche to return to your old meat-eating ways. Eaten with abandon, red meat can throw your dinner plate off balance, fatwise. Eaten in moderation, however, lean red meat can actually complement a low-fat, low-cholesterol diet. In addition to the nutritional advantages mentioned above, a little meat can add a depth of flavor to dishes that vegetables alone can't provide. Asian stir-fries and certain Italian sauces, for instance, draw astonishing flavor from the few ounces of lean red meat in each serving.

So, meat lovers, take heart: Modest portions of beef, pork and lamb (3½ ounces) served about two or three times a week won't blow your fat budget.

With proper planning and preparation, a meal with meat can contain less than 25 percent of calories from fat—a level many consider optimum for preventing heart disease and even cancer.

Following are some suggestions to help you prepare red meat to its best (health) advantage.

Shopping for the Leanest Cuts

Good news! Supermarket red meat has been sent to the commercial fat farm. More and more meat retailers are trimming their beef of excess fat. A quarter-inch seems to be the new standard. That means you're not paying for a lot of excess fat that you have to remove when you get home. And it's easier to shave off what's left.

Shoppers are getting wise, too—to the difference between grades of meat. The USDA grades meat Prime, Choice or Select according to the amount of fat marbling it contains. Marbling refers to the nonremovable, intramuscular fat that gives meat a grainy appearance; the more marbling, the more tender, flavorful and juicy the meat— but the more fat it contains.

Making the grade isn't the only thing that's important; the meat you choose should be a leaner cut. Fat content varies widely depending on where it comes from—the ribs, loin or rump, for example. (For the leanest cuts, see "How the Cuts Stack Up," on page 101.)

Preparing Lean Meat for Cooking

Trim it. Even the leanest cut isn't lean enough to cook without some prudent pruning. Be sure to trim all visible fat from meat before cooking. To simplify the task, place the meat in the freezer until partially frozen, about 20 minutes. Even hidden fat will turn white when chilled, making it easier to spot and trim with a sharp knife.

Marinate it. Some lean cuts, like flank steak or London broil, may benefit from this tenderizing technique. The secret to marinating is to soak the meat in an acidic solution before cooking. For best results use a marinade recipe that contains an acidic ingredient, such as yogurt, vinegar or citrus juice. This not only adds flavor but also can help break down the meat fibers to make it more palatable. A flavorful blend might include defatted beef stock, low-sodium soy sauce, lemon juice and herbs. Allow the meat to marinate in the refrigerator for several hours or overnight.

Cooking the Lean Cuts

There are two basic methods of cooking lean cuts; neither method uses added fat. The first method allows the fat from the meat to drain away. Examples of this method are stove-top grilling, broiling and roasting.

The other techniques still cook meat with no added fat. Although these methods do not permit the fat from the meat to drain away, with extremely lean cuts and reduced portion sizes, the additional fat is negligible. Examples of this method are braising, clay cooking and stir-frying.

When using one of the first three methods, you can prevent the meat from drying out during cooking by basting periodically with low-sodium broth or soy sauce, or pineapple juice. Or brush meat with reserved marinade that's been heated to a boil (after the raw meat has been removed) to kill any bacteria.

Stove-top grilling. This relatively fast method is good for cuts that are no more than one inch thick. It gives meat a crisp exterior and a juicy interior. You can take your choice of equipment: a ridged cast-iron grill pan or one of the new stove-top grill pans that work with water.

To use either piece of equipment, heat the pan until splashed on drops of cold water jump. Press the meat flat on the grill. For extra moistness, brush the meat with marinade as it cooks.

Broiling. In broiling, meat cooks directly under the flame or electric element. Position the pan so the meat is three to five inches from the heat source. Use a broiling rack and a drip pan. To retain moistness, brush the meat with marinade occasionally.

Roasting. Butchers recommend roasting larger, thicker cuts of meat by dry heat in a medium (350°F) oven. By tenderizing the fibers as the meat cooks, roasting can soften even inexpensive and low-fat cuts. Be sure to use a roasting rack or "meat feet" so fat can drain away. Roasted meats develop a crispy, browned exterior and a tender, juicy interior. As with broiling and grilling, basting the meat with a fat-free marinade gives tasty results.

Braising. Braised meat is browned, then simmered in liquid. It's often done in a Dutch oven and can take a good hour or more. It's a great way to tenderize lean cuts.

Clay cooking. Clay cookers act like mini-ovens that seal in moisture, allowing for slow, even cooking. Before cooking, submerge both the pot and its lid in cold water for five minutes. Then add your ingredients, cover and place the pot in a cold oven. Do not preheat the oven or the clay pot might crack. After cooking, allow the cooker to cool completely before washing. Use hot water and no detergent—the clay would absorb it and release it into food.

Stir-frying. The favored method of Asian cooks, stir-frying gives tough cuts of meat another chance. Marinate them first, then cook over high heat to retain moisture. Steam-stirring is a cousin of stir-frying. Sear the meat, then add a small amount of liquid, cover the pan and steam the meat until tender.

Reproportioning the Dinner Plate

Stop thinking of meat as the star of your meals. Regard it instead as an ensemble player, sharing equal billing with vegetables, grains and condiments. Keep in mind that a

How the Cuts Stack Up

It can be awfully confusing to sort out the various cuts of meat available in supermarkets, especially since many go by different names in different places.

The following cuts are good choices because they're low in fat. The numbers represent average values for three ounces of cooked meat (four ounces, trimmed, before cooking). If you have trouble identifying these cuts in the market, ask the person behind the meat counter for help.

Meat (3 oz.)	Fat (g)	Calories
Beef ◆		
Eye of round, roast	4.2	143
Top round, steak or roast	4.2	153
Tip round, steak or roast	5.9	157
Top sirloin, steak or roast	6.1	165
Top loin, steak	8.0	176
Tenderloin	8.5	179
Flank, steak	8.6	176
Pork ◆		
Tenderloin	4.1	141
Center loin, roast	8.9	196
Lamb ◆		
Leg, shank	5.7	153
Loin, chop or roast	7.8	173
Sirloin, chop or roast	7.8	173

healthful serving of meat is no more than 3½ ounces. Use a kitchen scale to help you learn what that amount looks like. If dealing with a steak or roast, three ounces of cooked meat is the size of a deck of playing cards. To "stretch" your portions, try the following tips.

Cut and fan. Slice the meat very thinly, especially on a diagonal across the grain. Then fan the slices out on a plate to give the illusion of a big serving.

Serve on a bed of wild greens. Instead of serving a large steak with a small, pale green salad on the side, take a tip from the Europeans; toss a generous assortment of greens like arugula, endive, raddichio and fresh herbs, top with a few slices of grilled meat (still warm) and drizzle the salad with balsamic vinegar.

Make a mostly vegetable stew, stir-fry, kabob or casserole. Serve over a heaping mound of rice, bulgur or couscous.

CHAPTER

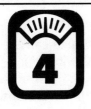

ENERGIZE WITH EXERCISE: HOW FITNESS CAN BOOST FAT LOSS

Welcome to the brave new world of fitness. The good news is that exercise has changed a lot since calisthenics and your high school gym class! The following articles are gleaned from this year's newest, most exciting exercise research to help you change the way you think about working out.

How 10 Popular Exercises Rate as Fat Burners
By Covert Bailey

Nutritional biochemist, head of the Bailey Fit-or-Fat Center in Oregon, lecturer and leader of nationwide seminars

Diets alone are not, and never have been, an effective way to lose weight and keep it off. Diets don't attack the fundamental problem of the overweight person, which is that his or her metabolism tends to burn up fewer calories and store more of them as fat.

The only permanent cure for obesity is aerobic exercise. It builds muscle, tones it, alters its chemistry and increases its metabolic rate. All of these processes cause you to burn more calories, even when you're asleep.

Listed below is the long-term fat-burning potential of ten popular exercises. You'll probably notice that in most but not all cases, exercises that have high fat-burning potential also carry a greater risk of injury. Any exercise that is weight-bearing, uses a lot of different muscle groups and involves bouncing and jarring of joints is bound to have victims.

Running, one of the fastest fat-burning exercises, has gotten somewhat of a tarnished reputation from the growing list of runners who sustain injuries. But a closer look at statistics reveals that the majority of these injuries occur in those who run more than 35 miles a week.

Whatever you do, don't focus your fat-burning program on just one exercise. If you do, you'll either become totally bored and stop exercising or you'll hurt yourself. If possible, cross-train, varying your exercise routine among three or four favorites. If you especially enjoy doing one of the exercises that has a higher risk of injury, that's fine. Just don't overdo it. The following list shows that you can add high-fat-burning but low-injury-risk activities to your program without sacrificing the quality of your workout.

Outdoor Exercises

Cross-Country Skiing
Long-term fat-burning potential: very high
Injury risk: low
Cross-country skiing is the fastest fat burner and is more strenuous than running, yet has a low risk of injury because its movements are gliding rather than bouncing. The start-up costs are fairly low compared to those of downhill skiing, and you can experiment with rental equipment. I recommend cross-country skiing for people who are already in pretty good shape. It's a deceptive exercise in that it requires skill and balance along with good arm and leg coordination. You'll be surprised how tiring it can be, even though your pace is usually slower than your jogging/running pace.

Cross-country skiing is no longer seasonal. There are several fine machines on the market that simulate the striding leg motion synchronized with arm and shoulder movement. There are also special ski skates available to help you stay in shape during summer months.

Running
Long-term fat-burning potential: high
Injury risk: moderate for mileages under 35 per week; very high over 35 miles per week

By far the best known aerobic exercise, jogging is one of the easiest programs to start. The only equipment you need is a pair of good running shoes. In general, most of you who haven't been in a running program will be classified as joggers. (There's controversy about this, but as a general rule of thumb, if it takes you more than eight minutes to travel a mile, you're jogging.)

The injury risk with jogging or running is mainly to joints, ligaments and muscles of the lower body. If you're plagued with knee, ankle or lower back pain, you can try varying the length of your stride, your speed or your foot strike. (A heel/ball step works best when running a mile in more than eight minutes.) If possible, run on softer surfaces such as wood-chip trails or rubberized asphalt. Do not persist if the pain doesn't let up in a day or two. Switch to another exercise, and be sure to have a doctor check out the problem.

Cycling
Long-term fat-burning potential: moderate

Injury risk: low from the sport itself but high if collisions and accidents are included

Cycling is the exercise you fall in love with. Because it uses fewer muscles than running and because it is not weight-bearing, you'll have to cycle about 40 minutes to equal 20 minutes of jogging. But most people don't mind at all. Bicycling is usually a joyful pastime rather than an exercise in drudgery. Moreover, when elite runners and cyclists are compared, cyclists, as a group, come out looking fitter. This is because the low injury rate among cyclists allows them to spend more time in training and less time in recovery.

Cycling does have drawbacks. It may not be easy to find nonstop routes so you can maintain a steady exercise pulse. Also, it's tricky learning to change gears so you can go smoothly up and down hills. Try to maintain a steady pace of about 70 revolutions a minute instead of bursts of pushing and coasting.

Walking

Long-term fat-burning potential: moderately low if total walking time is 30 minutes or less or walking speed is slower than 15 minutes a mile; moderate if more than 30 minutes or faster than 15 minutes a mile; high for race walking

Injury risk: low

Walking must be fairly vigorous to give fat-burning benefits. Try to set a pace of at least a hundred steps a minute and less than 20 minutes a mile. You have to walk for about 45 minutes to equal 20 minutes of jogging.

Race walking, or power walking, is rapidly gaining popularity, and I heartily applaud its proponents. The vigorous arm swinging and the odd hip movement that makes the power walker resemble a frantic duck really chews up the calories. Many race walkers can outpace joggers. I believe that after we get past the laughter, power walking is going to be the choice exercise of the future, giving a better workout with half the jarring impact of running.

Swimming

Long-term fat-burning potential: low

Injury risk: very low

Swimming is the most injury-free sport around. It gives excellent cardiovascular benefits and is great for toning practically all your muscles. But if you're overweight, I don't recommend it as your only exercise. Of the thousands of people I've tested for body fat, swimmers consistently carry more fat than runners or cyclists.

So, you can get very fit with swimming, but you probably won't lose much fat. Please note that I have not said swimming makes you fat, nor have I said that swimming does not decrease body fat. If you are 35 percent fat to start with, you will lose fat more slowly with swimming than with land sports. You will not get fatter. If you are lean and fit when you take up swimming, you will stay lean and fit, but your body fat will probably not decrease.

Despite this drawback, I think swimming is a good starting program for overweight people who are unused to exercise. They can learn body coordination and gain fitness without feeling clumsy or risking injury to already overburdened joints. Once they've built up a certain amount of coordination and fitness, they can venture on to exercises that burn more fat.

Indoor Exercises

You should try to find at least one indoor exercise for times when the weather is bad or your time is limited. I like to use indoor exercise equipment as an adjunct to outdoor activity.

Many of the following exercises require the purchase of some serious equipment. As a general rule of thumb, the heavier and more costly the machine, the better it is. If you get something cheap, it will probably end up as an expensive clothes rack in six months. It's best to try the equipment before purchasing.

Rowing Machine
Long-term fat-burning potential: high
Injury risk: low

Indoors or outdoors, rowing is a high fat-consuming exercise. Like cross-country skiing, it exercises most of the large muscle groups without stress on joints and has the added benefit of developing the muscles of the upper torso. It's one of the few aerobic exercises that can be performed with one leg if the other is injured.

Stair Climber
Long-term fat-burning potential: high
Injury risk: moderately low

This seemingly mild, low-impact exercise yields terrific fat-burning results. It's as energy demanding as running but with no more force to the joints than walking.

Way back when exercise testing was in its infancy, the chair-step test used to be the standard method for determining fitness. It was simple: You got an eight-inch-high stool, stepped up with the right foot, brought the left foot up, stepped down with the right foot, then brought the left foot down. If you did this for 15 minutes, you chalked up a fat-burning, cardiovascular-improving aerobic exercise for the day. This simple little exercise has now reaped millions of dollars for the manufacturers of stair-climbing machines.

The popularity of these machines is amazing. People have to make reservations days in advance to use one. Although they won't make you any more fit than climbing regular stairs, they do offer some pluses, such as variable resistance and continuous uphill work.

Jump Rope
Long-term fat-burning potential: high
Injury risk: moderately high

I think everyone should have a jump rope around, just in case. If you're a runner, it's great to use when you're traveling and prefer not to run in strange neighborhoods. You can keep a jump rope at work and use it instead of taking a 15-minute coffee break. I've even jumped rope up and down the aisle of a 747 during a long overseas flight.

Jumping rope is best as an alternative exercise for those days when time is limited or you'd rather stay indoors. It's a bit too strenuous and hard on joints to be used every day.

Treadmill

Long-term fat-burning potential: moderate to high, depending on incline and speed

Injury risk: low

A treadmill may be either self-powered or motorized. By changing the incline or the speed, you can power walk, run, or hike uphill. Many people find that they avoid the sore knees and back problems associated with jogging when they switch to a treadmill.

Your best pace on a treadmill is a fast walk or slow jog. Unfortunately, the macho instinct emerges, and I've seen many overweight and unconditioned men running at a pace that even a seasoned runner would find difficult to maintain. Use some sense with this machine. Go 15 steady fat-burning minutes at a moderate pace instead of 3 panting anaerobic minutes of heart-stopping hell.

Stationary Bicycle

Long-term fat-burning potential: moderate

Injury risk: low

I like stationary bicycling because I can do two things at once. While I'm exercising, I can read a book or watch the evening news. There are even bike videos available for those of you who prefer a scenic route during your indoor exercise. You can even try weight lifting while using a stationary bicycle. You can pedal while pumping light weights overhead to strengthen shoulders, do biceps curls, triceps back extensions and frontal flys for the pectorals.

Why Work Out?
By Phil Dunphy

Physical therapist, exercise physiologist and former owner of HEAR (Health through Exercise and Rehabilitation)

The fact that you're reading this shows that you have a steady interest in gaining or maintaining better health through exercise. But now it's time to move up a step in fitness awareness.

Don't worry, we won't bury you in needless details. Think of it as the sort of review you might have gotten at school when you returned from summer vacation. More than anything, we're going to remind you of things you really do know but haven't thought of in a while: the benefits of exercise.

1. You'll look better! By losing fat weight and gaining muscle, your clothes will fit better and allow you to expand your wardrobe into the fashions of the 1990s (or at least the 1980s!). Clothes don't make the person; the person who exercises makes the clothes!

2. Your sex life will improve. Research has shown that those who exercise have better sex. No surprise. Sexual activity is physical, and it requires energy, muscle control and a high degree of sensitivity. You can't be very sensitive if you're out of breath and don't like the way your body looks.

3. You will be doing your heart a big favor. Heaps of studies have shown over and over again that exercise improves your "heart health." It can cut your cholesterol and triglyceride levels, raise your HDL (good) cholesterol and lower your blood pressure into the normal range.

4. You will fight the aging process. The ability of your muscles and other tissues to utilize oxygen (called

◆

max VO$_2$) decreases naturally as you age. But exercise can slow the rate of this loss.

Basal metabolic rate (the rate at which we burn calories at rest) also drops as we get older. You can easily gain ten pounds of fat per year as you age—even though your activity level and calorie intake stay the same—because your metabolism is slowing down. But exercise can compensate. Regular workouts can keep us moving along, helping us to burn more calories. And that benefit carries over from exercise to increased calorie burn even while we rest!

5. You'll be making the best of aging when it does catch up. Bones, muscles and the fibers that tie them together work better when they're used. Exercise can help to prevent injuries—today or tomorrow.

But it's even more important to plan for long-term health by concentrating on standing up straight, keeping the head back atop the shoulders and maintaining strong, flexible muscles. The simple fact is that most of us are going to live longer than our parents. And exercise can help us enjoy rather than suffer through our later years. If we keep our bodies fit, we can stay independent and active and age gracefully.

6. Exercise and eating go together. It's not just that you need proper nutrition to develop physically. You need exercise to complement your eating habits. The data are in, and all the studies show that sitting around and starving ourselves is not the ticket to health. Eating more of the right stuff and exercising more is the better path.

Exercise must be included in a successful nutrition program to keep weight off and get the most out of life. Exercise helps you process your food, and it allows you a high enough calorie intake to ensure proper nutrition—without putting on weight.

7. You'll feel better about yourself. Once you start dropping a few pounds, fitting into more flattering clothes and building some good muscles, you'll start to feel more confident, not only about your appearance but about your abilities and lots of other things in your life. Add a few compliments from others to the equation, and pretty soon you'll be feeling better about life than you may have in a while.

So there you are. Seven reasons why exercise is as fundamental to life as eating and sleeping. There are many more, but these points cover some of the most important reasons for exercise. It's a good idea to remind yourself of these reasons to help you keep in perspective what you're trying to accomplish with a fitness program. The goals determine the methods. And well-rounded goals ensure a well-rounded program.

Reprogram Your Metabolism to Burn More Fat

Metabolism can be your body's built-in weight-loss plan. When it's fired up, it gobbles calories like a party crasher at a buffet spread. When it's lazy, it just nibbles and then yawns.

Resistance training kicks this process into high gear. It boosts your metabolism's appetite and eggs it on to burn more calories. This in turn may help you maximize your health in three powerful ways:

- By losing weight without sacrificing valuable muscle
- By putting a heart-healthy shine on your cholesterol profile
- By helping to control diabetes through improving the way your body metabolizes glucose and deals with insulin

A charged-up metabolism boosts these processes by adding muscle and subtracting fat. This change in body composition—brought on by resistance training—is what gets the metabolic action in high gear.

Burn by Building

Imagine pumping the accelerator of an idling car—it burns more gas even though it's in park. Resistance training does the same thing—you burn more calories even when you're in park. It's a pumping irony: Though the amount of calories burned during resistance training isn't as large when compared to aerobic workouts such as running, over the long haul the extra muscle you gain may mean a potential for more calorie burning. Why? Because muscle is active tissue; fat is inactive.

"You can spend 40 minutes weight training and maybe burn 150 calories, which isn't that much compared to aerobic exercise," says Janet Walberg-Rankin, Ph.D., associate professor at Virginia Tech. "But lean muscle tissue is more metabolically active than fat tissue; it needs more calories. Since resistance training creates more muscle, you build more tissue that needs calories. If you increase muscle mass while you lose fat, you boost your ability to burn calories."

Even though during strength training the calories aren't shedding quickly, it's later in the day, when you're relaxing or waiting in line at the bank, that your new, improved metabolic rate is grinding away. The change in body composition—more muscle and less fat—means hungrier tissue. The more ravenous muscle you have, the more you may be able to eat and the more energy you can burn.

Now there's no question aerobic exercise should always be part of the battle plan when you want to lose weight—it helps burn calories fast during the actual workout. But when you bolster this strategy with resistance training, the battle plan goes ballistic.

Igniting the Afterburn

In a study at Oregon Health Sciences University, researchers found that a group of exercisers who hit the weights ended up burning more calories afterward than those people who did aerobic exercise. The muscle builders had roused a hungrier caloric afterburn that devoured one-third more calories than the afterburn from aerobic exercise.

"The afterburn isn't that large and lasts 30 to 60 minutes, which adds up to about an extra one to two pounds a year lost if you exercise three times a week," says Linn Goldberg, M.D., one of the study researchers. "That's nothing to laugh at—most Americans gain one to two pounds a year. If the afterburn can offset that, that's great."

Add Weight and Lose It

When you drop a few pounds, make it fat. Adding strength work to an exercise program means losing the stuff you want to lose—the flab—and keeping the stuff that enables you to lug books, pick up kids and throw Frisbees—the muscle.

In one study, one group of obese women exercised both aerobically and with weight training four times a week (while on a very low-calorie diet). They ended up losing more fat while maintaining more of the fat-free mass than another group who only exercised aerobically. In the aerobics-only group, 76 percent of the body weight lost was fat, while it was 86 percent in the aerobics-plus-muscle-building group.

Resistance training may even reverse the muscle wasting that tends to occur when you're dieting. In another study, a group of obese women using strength training while dieting were able to lose the desired weight while actually increasing their muscle. They gained over one pound of muscle while another group dieting without strength training lost nearly three pounds of muscle.

Metabolic Motivation

The change in body composition can also muscle up the psyche. "With weight training, you get quick feedback—you can visually see the results," says Dr. Walberg-Rankin. "That can spur you on to continue your efforts in weight control."

Pushing the Cholesterol Plow

For improvements in cholesterol levels, muscle may do some very good deeds. Studies suggest that strength training may increase the good kind of cholesterol, HDL, while others show that it may tackle the bad blood fats (LDL cholesterol and triglycerides).

Reworking your body composition is key. "The rise in HDL cholesterol brought on by regular exercise may not be that great, unless a change in body composition occurs," says Dr. Goldberg. "Which is what resistance training helps to accomplish—by increasing muscle mass and decreasing fat."

In one of Dr. Goldberg's studies, eight women and six men participated in 16 weeks of weight training, exercising three days a week for 45 to 60 minutes. For the women, the ratio of total cholesterol to HDL cholesterol was reduced 14.3 percent after the program, with the LDL-to-HDL ratio also dropping 20.3 percent. Among men, the same ratios dropped 21.6 percent and 28.9 percent respectively. These ratios are potent predictors of heart disease—the lower the ratios the lower the risk.

"Even if the benefits from resistance training are only short-term, by exercising regularly you may be able to string together the temporary benefits into a long-term one," says Irma H. Ullrich, M.D., professor of medicine in the Section of Endocrinology and Metabolism at West Virginia University Medical Center. "But it's like taking medication—once you stop taking it, you end up back at square one." The researcher has seen resistance training's benefits up close. She conducted a study of 25 men who weight trained three times a week for eight weeks. Their HDL levels climbed from 38.8 to 44.1 mg/dl, with their LDLs dropping from 132 to 121.

Pump Down Diabetes

Resistance training may help improve the body's ability to process sugar properly. Now even more diabetes research is going beyond the lab and setting up shop in the gym.

Type-I Muscles

In a first-time study, researchers looked at the effects of resistance training on people with Type-I diabetes, who are dependent on insulin to metabolize their blood sugar.

Besides observing strength increases in the subjects after several weeks of heavy weight lifting, the researchers saw a drop in cholesterol and a decrease in "glycosylated hemoglobin," a marker for long-term elevations of glucose levels—suggesting that these men were able to keep their blood sugar under proper control over time.

"If a diabetic keeps that measurement low, we believe that as he gets older he may not develop retinopathy, kidney problems, impotence and other complications that occur from having diabetes," says Eric Durak, one of the authors of the study.

The cholesterol drop is another bonus, since blood sugar problems may interfere with the metabolism of cholesterol, Durak says. And since people with diabetes are often at increased risk for heart disease, the cholesterol drop is that much more important.

More Muscle, Less Insulin

Resistance training may also help to improve insulin sensitivity, so less insulin is needed to respond to sugar in the blood. After a 12-week weight-training program, six young and nine elderly healthy men all showed reductions in insulin response (a 43 percent drop in the young group, a 13 percent decline in the older). There ended up being less unused insulin in the blood.

"Their tissues picked up more glucose at the same rate with a reduced level of insulin," says B. W. Craig, Ph.D., associate director of exercise science at Ball State University. "The level of insulin goes down, and what insulin there is ends up being more effective. People with diabetes may be able to reduce their insulin intake and still handle their glucose more effectively."

These benefits followed a change in body composition—fat loss and muscle gain. "If you have a lot of fat, that tends to shut off your utilization of glucose. The fat is metabolized instead of the sugar," says Dr. Craig. "If you have more muscle, you have a greater ability to store glycogen. That helps improve metabolism of sugar," he says. Muscles become portable glucose bins—the larger the bin, the more space you have to take up glucose and store it as glycogen.

See Your Doctor, Check Your Levels

If you want to strength train and happen to be diabetic, see your doctor beforehand for a full evaluation. Also, "when you start your exercise program, monitor your blood glucose levels frequently throughout the workout just to see how they respond," says Dr. Craig. "That way you can adjust according to the changes." It's also important to get your eyes tested regularly. The jumps in blood pressure can be dangerous if you have ocular pressure problems.

Put the Muscle on Fat
By Phil Dunphy

Exercise doesn't only help us sweat off pounds and build muscle, it also is the secret ingredient in our war against fat.

Muscle Is the Engine

Muscle makes us work. It lifts our limbs, moves our eyes and pumps our blood. Muscle comes in two basic types:

- Slow-twitch muscles are good for endurance. They have lots of blood flow and make good use of oxygen.
- Fast-twitch muscles are good for short bursts of energy. They can utilize energy very quickly, but they have little endurance.

Like engines, muscles need fuel to work, and our two types of muscles have definite preferences.

Fat Is the Fuel

Fat is the predominant fuel in our bodies. Each of us stores enough of it to keep our muscle engine running all the way from New York City to Madison, Wisconsin. By contrast, the other significant fuel—carbohydrate—has a pretty tiny tank. Your carbo stores wouldn't get you beyond Passaic—a mere 20 miles.

Although both types of muscle can utilize fat or carbohydrate, slow-twitch muscles are much better at handling fat, and fast-twitch muscles do really well with carbos. When you think about it, it makes perfect sense. The endurance muscles use the biggest store of energy.

Once you understand that, it's easy to see why you've got to work out moderately over an extended period to burn fat efficiently. Only the slow-twitch muscles do a good job of using it. If you beat the heck out of your body, your fast-twitch muscles will do most of the work. You'll burn up a bunch of carbos—but very little fat.

Why Dieting Alone Won't Work

If you've tried dieting alone, you know this basic truth: At some point in your dieting, you hit a point where you can't seem to lose the last of your flab, no matter how much you deprive yourself of food. That's because, as you've lost weight, you've also lost muscle. Your metabolic rate—the rate you burn fuel—has dropped because your engine has gotten smaller. To lose more fat, you need to build muscle.

Here's an illustration of just how significant muscles really are in the metabolic picture. Even when you're asleep, your muscles use up 25 percent of the energy you burn. And the more muscle you have, the more energy you burn.

So you begin to see that exercise can help you shed fat in several different ways:

1. As you build bigger muscles, your metabolic rate goes up. You burn more calories no matter what you're doing: running, walking, mowing the lawn, reading the paper, even sleeping.

2. A properly designed exercise program can burn fat directly.

3. And even the parts of your workout that burn carbohydrates are helpful. At least those calories aren't hanging around waiting to become fat.

How Much Fat Is Good?

Some fat is absolutely necessary to health. Not only does it provide the major endurance energy source, but it cushions internal organs and carries the fat-soluble vitamins (A, E and the carotenoids) to places where they're needed.

But most people carry too much. Somewhere in the vicinity of 15 to 16 percent of total body weight in fat is about right for most men. For women, that percent is a little higher; between 18 and 22 percent is considered ideal for young women. Basically, any more than those percentages is going to be carried under your skin as adipose. But be encouraged. Those percentages can go up a bit as you age.

Add Variety to Burn More Calories in Walks
By Ralph LaForge

Teacher of exercise physiology at the University of California, San Diego, and director of Health Promotion at the San Diego Cardiac Center Medical Group

Walking is the simplest, least stressful aerobic exercise you can do. It carries little risk of injury. It can be done just about anywhere, at almost anytime.

When done regularly and vigorously, walking benefits your body in important ways: improved heart and lung functioning, toned up and strong muscles, relaxation, relief from stress and loss of unwanted pounds.

Furthermore, walking is adaptable. In the beginning when muscles are flaccid and untrained, walk at a slow to normal pace, for short periods of time. As your stamina improves, speed up the pace gradually and walk for an hour or longer.

Slow Down and Walk Farther

I've worked with Type A persons—always rushed because of meetings, projects, deadlines—who tend to allocate their time. Walking may rate a 20-minute slot during which Mr. or Ms. Type A sets forth as fast as possible. That technique is neither efficient at burning calories nor at relieving stress. If your goal is to lose weight, you'll want to know that you actually burn more calories when you slow down slightly and walk farther over hilly terrain. In a program I developed for the San Diego Police Department, officers were more successful at losing weight when they did variable-terrain walking.

The Surprising Power of Hills

Variable-terrain walking—over hills and through valleys—burns up to 25 percent more calories, on average, than walking over flat terrain. And you need not push yourself. A rate of about three miles per hour is sufficient.

In fact, the safest and most effective cardio-respiratory weight control exercise for those who are 20 to 30 pounds overweight is progressive variable-terrain walking.

How to Begin Variable-Terrain Walking

1. Shoes are important. Specialized walking shoes are fine, although in my experience, many walkers prefer a good pair of running shoes.

2. Always warm up and cool down. Begin each session by walking for about five minutes, then stretch your Achilles tendon, calf and lower back muscles. After your walk, cool down by walking at a slower pace, then again stretch the muscles mentioned above.

3. When you first begin your walking program, work on duration—the length of time you walk. Start with a 15-minute walk, or one mile. Work up to a 60-minute walk.

Then gradually add faster-paced walking or intensity. Adding hilly terrain also adds intensity. When you travel over routes with hills, remember to slow down a bit. A pace of 20 minutes per mile is fine.

Over Hill, Over Dale

Adding the variety of hilly terrain can give you a change of scenery, which is always a plus. It certainly beats riding a stationary bicycle for an hour in front of the television set.

Map out a variety of locations to walk in order to build muscular strength and endurance. For the most benefit, don't walk the same ten-block route near your house every day. When your plantar, or foot, muscles adapt to a terrain—say, the floor of your house—they are not challenged and become lazy.

Here is a suggested weekly routine to get you started.

Several days per week: Walk your usual course. Change the direction of your walk so the terrain varies somewhat from day to day.

Once weekly: Walk on a high school track and really push for speed. (This is great for mothers with toddlers. Let them play on the grass inside the track while you exercise.)

Once or twice weekly: Walk on the trails of a public park or access paths of a public golf course at dawn or dusk.

On the weekend: Take a canteen of water and walk in the country. Treat yourself to an hour or two of hiking; this longer walk confers fitness that you don't get during the work week.

Reprinted with permission from *Executive Health's Good Health Report,* July 1991.

Pool Walking Is Making a Splash

Walking in the pool burns calories while it relieves stress and strengthens muscles. Water gives ten times the resistance of air, and your muscles get a working over in two directions—as you extend your legs and when you push off.

Begin by walking forward and then try going backward and sideways. You'll find some muscles you didn't know about before. As a bonus, being in the water reduces the compressive forces of gravity on your muscles, joints and bones. If you like what pool walking can do for your body, check if your gym or local college offers classes in water aerobics, too.

A Better Back and a Stronger Stomach, All in One!

Most people firm up their stomachs so they'll look good in a swimsuit, and there's nothing wrong with trimming your tummy for the beach. But one surefire strategy to help slim your stomach can also improve your body in another, more important way—by bolstering your back and preventing low back pain, which many of us know is all too common when you're overweight. The strategy is exercise. The very exercises that home in on the abdominal muscles end up giving a healthy boost to the skeletal support center of your body—your lower back.

Backing into Benefits

Chances are you don't think much about your back until you're forced to—when you feel that first pulse of pain after helping a friend move an antique trunk into her apartment, or just lifting your two-year-old son. The fact is, when it comes to back pain, a weak abdomen can usually be spotted at the scene of the crime. Back specialists have known this for years.

When researchers look at people with low back pain, they often find abdominal muscles are much weaker than the low back muscles. One study looked at healthy people and those with back pain and found no difference in back-muscle endurance. Stomach-muscle endurance, however, was much less in the group with pain. In short, much back pain may not be simply due to weak back muscles—the culprit may lurk on the other side of the trunk.

In the 1940s, when Hans Kraus, M.D., an internationally known back specialist, found a strong correlation between weak stomach muscles and back pain, he incorporated abdominal exercises into a back strategy that eventually became the YMCA Healthy Back Program. And it worked. In one evaluation of 233 patients who took part in the program, 82 percent found that their usual back pain was either prevented or significantly reduced. Another 15 percent had a fair response, and only 2.5 percent showed little or no improvement.

"In our program we stress flexibility, relaxation and abdominal strength," says Michael Spezzano, former national director of the YMCA Healthy Back Program and YMCA fitness specialist. "The abdominal exercises are painless and easy to do, and they work."

The fact that a strong abdomen helps your back has been accepted as anatomically obvious. Major back clinics, including the Texas Back Institute (TBI) and the YMCA program, include abdominal strengthening exercises in their programs, along with other exercises and stretches that target the back.

Specifically, here's how building strong stomach muscles can help bolster your back.

Building a Firmer Foundation

We all worry about what's behind us, and yet most of us don't even know what the muscles in our buttocks are called. They are the gluteal muscles, some of the largest yet most often neglected muscles in our bodies. Here are a few of the best exercises you can do for a shapely, lower half.

1. Alternated front lunge. Keep your head up, your back straight and your feet 14 inches apart. Step forward as far as possible with your right leg until the upper right thigh is almost parallel to the floor. Keep your lower leg straight. Step back to the starting position. Repeat with the left leg. This can also be done with a light weight, holding it straight down at the sides. You can try it next to a chair; hold on to the back of the chair to help maintain balance.

2. Kneeling back kick. Kneel with your left knee on a bench. Hold the outer sides of the bench, keeping your arms locked. Let your right leg hang down. Raise your right leg straight back as far as you can (keeping the leg straight). Return to the starting position and then repeat with your left leg.

3. Freehand jump squat. Stand with your arms crossed over your chest. Keep your head up, with your back straight and your feet roughly 16 inches apart. Squat until your upper thighs are parallel with the floor. Jump straight up in the air as high as you can. Immediately squat and repeat the jump.

Abs Stabilize the Spine

Developing the abdominal and back muscles to their highest potential helps keep the spine in a neutral position. "The abdominal muscles and the low back muscles together form a column of muscles that must be strong all around," says Wayne Westcott, Ph.D., YMCA National

Strength Training Consultant, from Quincy, Massachusetts. "If one side is weak, it's going to put excess stress on the spine and the nerves and tissue that surround it."

Eventually the stress caused by weak abdominal muscles can lead to excessive lordosis (often called swayback) of the lumbar (lower) spine, increasing the potential risk for spinal injuries. If back and stomach muscles are made stronger, however, the load that the spine has to support is decreased.

Weak abs can be made worse—with a knife and fork. "For Americans the abdomen is the weak link, because it's exercised very little and it's where body fat tends to migrate," says Dr. Westcott. It's a double whammy—like sending extra traffic to a congested bridge with weak supports. Something's got to give. In this case, it's your spine. A potbelly on top of weak ab muscles creates an effect much like a pregnant woman experiences when carrying her umbilicaled house guest—the large imbalance creates a swayback (excessive inward curving of the spine). "That's why a healthy diet is just as important for your back as strong abdominal muscles are," says Dr. Westcott.

"The last thing your spine needs to support is a big belly." A low-fat diet coupled with a full exercise program that emphasizes abdominal work may be as close as you can get to natural liposuction for a potbelly. People who put away more than two drinks a day will do well to cut back. Excess alcohol, it seems, adds flab to that pot.

Strong Abs Balance Your Back

A strong abdomen helps the body deal with resistive force, whether it's moving furniture or participating in an activity like catching a ball. "If those abdominal muscles are weak, you'll overcompensate with your back," says Paula Gilbert, physical therapist at the TBI. "This can lead to a back sprain over and over again. You need to have these stomach and back muscles synergized—working together—or your back will not respond well after injury."

Working the Abs Gives a Relaxing Reflex

While exercising the stomach, you're giving your back on-the-spot relief. "Working the muscles in a crunch sit-up gives a slight stretch to the back muscles," says Gilbert. "This gives you a reflex relaxation of the back extensor muscles, so you feel better after doing the exercises."

When you lie on the floor with your knees up, in the sit-up position, there's a normal arch in your back—what's called the normal lumbar curve. "The movement from the sit-up reverses that normal curve," says Dr. Westcott. "As you curl your shoulders and head off the floor, your lower back presses into the floor. The lower back is now being stretched, which it so desperately needs because often it's too tight." By lying on the floor, your lower back is also being stretched safely with support.

Say No to One-Spot Fitness

Now we know why a strong abdomen makes perfect body sense. Remember, though, that zeroing in on your stomach muscles, while neglecting other aspects of fitness, makes almost no sense. Here's why.

"You need to increase all components of physical fitness, especially cardiovascular fitness, to decrease back pain and injury," says Gilbert. "Walking, swimming, water exercises or stationary cycling keeps your body flexible and fit and thus helps prevent you from overworking your back."

"It's like lubricating oil for the spine," says Stephen Hochschuler, M.D., surgeon and cofounder of TBI, and author of the book *Back in Shape.* "Cardiovascular exercise lubricates the joints and stretches muscles so they are less prone to strain and tearing." Cardiovascular exercise keeps the oxygen level up in your bloodstream, helping the muscles work in a more efficient fashion. "You develop a transport system to get oxygen into the tissues. It helps with healing in case your back does get injured," says Gilbert.

A study of 1,652 firefighters shows that inactivity can fan the flames of back pain. Researchers looked at the frequency of back injuries among the least and most cardiovascularly fit. Seven percent of the least fit had back injuries intense enough to call in sick for work—an amount ten times greater than those who were the most physically fit. And when the most fit firefighters did suffer a back injury, they also recovered faster and returned to work sooner than those injured in the least-fit group.

"Back pain, like cardiovascular disease, can be a lifestyle disease," says Mitch Bogdanffy, an exercise physiologist at TBI. "In many of the patients we see, back pain turns out to be a symptom caused by a life of inactivity."

Resistance exercises can specifically target back muscles, while weight-bearing exercises like walking also provide a boost. "Walking pumps the back muscles, increasing their endurance so they can withstand the pressure when you're picking something up or just being on your feet eight hours a day," says Gilbert. Strengthening leg muscles, which share lifting duty with the back, is also key. Strong leg muscles, by taking most of the burden of lifting, prevent the back muscles from binding up or going into spasms under heavy loads. Leg flexibility is another important aspect, so you need to do leg stretches as part of your daily back regimen. And needless to say, having strong arms means less work for the back when you're lifting a small child or tossing a football. Resistance training can hit all these spots.

And remember, daily exercise boosts the production of your own self-made painkillers, the endorphins and enkephalins, which may also take a bite out of back pain.

Tummy Tips

Before you hit the floor and work your abs, here are a few tips to get you on your way to a stronger back.

If you have a serious back problem, see an orthopedist or physical therapist before undertaking any exercise program. "Most people with back pain can do light exercises," says Gilbert. "But if you can't find any position that gives you relief or if simple movement makes the pain worse, then you need to see a doctor." And remember, too, that serious back pain isn't always due to muscle weakness.

Use your built-in equipment. When doing stomach-muscle exercises, all the resistance equipment you need is at your fingertips—or at least connected to them: your limbs. "When you do these exercises, you can move your legs much like levers," says Dr. Westcott. "You're changing your center of gravity to add to the difficulty. Your body provides the resistance. You don't need weights."

For example, instead of doing all your sit-ups in the standard position (feet flat on the floor, knees bent) try elevating your legs off the ground, so that your legs are straight up in the air, or bent in the air. Also, try moving your knees toward your elbows and raising your hips a bit off the floor as you come up into the sit-up.

Keep it slow. When it comes to speed for abdominal exercises, less is more. "You don't need to do hundreds of sit-ups real fast to have an effect," says Dr. Westcott. "Abdominal muscles are small. Slow, controlled movements of up to ten repetitions per exercise is all you need, and you'll have better results." Don't rely on momentum. "When you do them fast, the momentum carries you, and the stomach muscles end up doing less work," he says.

Stay low. You don't have to go all the way up. "When you do a full sit-up, you use only about 30 percent of the abdominal muscles. The hip flexors are doing most of the work," says Dr. Westcott. "If you do a crunch sit-up, in which you go up slightly, with just your head and shoulders coming up off the ground, you end up using the right muscles to do 90 percent of the work."

And don't go loco. Get to know your tolerance level slowly. "Start out with one exercise at a time, and add another new exercise when you feel up to it," says Gilbert. You can start with six to eight repetitions per exercise. As they become easier you can do more. These exercises and at least a short walk should become a daily habit, like brushing your teeth.

Get vain. Try doing the exercises in front of a mirror and check your body position as you work out.

Get a mat. Put something between you and the floor. A body-length mat cushions your back much better than a cold, hard floor.

Hands off! Don't place your hands behind your neck when you're doing a sit-up. "People have a tendency to pull on their neck and strain it," says exercise physiologist Daniel Foster, who specializes in strength training and is coordinator of research programs and services at the Center for Exercise Science, University of Florida at Gainesville. "Place your hands across your chest or, if you want your hands up by your neck, don't clasp them."

Oblige the obliques. The obliques are the abdominal side muscles and are as important as any of the other trunk muscles. "Applying a slight twist toward one knee with the opposite arm when you come up slowly on a sit-up works your obliques effectively," says Dr. Westcott.

Rotate and tilt. "The pelvic tilt is a relatively easy exercise that takes the stress off the back," says Bogdanffy. "When you contract your abdomen and rotate your pelvis back, you take stress off the lumbar disks."

Get creative. The abdomen wasn't created just to do abdominal exercises. Working the muscles can be a by-product of having fun. "Yoga, dancing and t'ai chi ch'uan are great ways to strengthen the stomach muscles in a dynamic way," says Gilbert.

Exercises for Your Front and Back

1. Pelvic tilt. Lie on your back on the floor, with your knees raised and arms extended. Press your lower back down against the floor by tightening the abdominal muscles, squeezing the buttocks and rolling the top of the pelvis backward. Hold for a few seconds and repeat.

2. Partial curl (or crunch). Lie on your back with your knees bent. Extend your hands between your thighs. Slowly curl your upper torso until your shoulder blades leave the floor. Hold a few seconds, go down and repeat. Exhale as you rise.

3. Advanced curl. Lie on your back with your knees bent and your fingers lightly touching your ears. Slowly curl your upper torso until your shoulders leave the floor. Hold a few seconds; inhale as you go back down.

4. Twist curl. Lie on the floor with your knees bent. Fold your arms across your chest. Slowly curl your right shoulder off the floor toward your left knee until your left shoulder leaves the floor. Hold for a few seconds, breathing deeply. Repeat, but with your left shoulder toward your right knee.

Dance! A New Twist on Fitness

What fitness activity takes the cooperation of four feet, four hands and two hearts, can be performed in public and is so much fun you forget you're exercising?

It's ballroom dancing, and it's on the upswing across the country, with folks doing everything from graceful waltzes to steamy sambas. What used to be considered purely a social pursuit is now being recognized as a fun way to fitness as well. Many people think the aerobic value of ballroom dancing lies somewhere between a slow-stepping waltz and spirited conversation. They don't realize that a waltzing couple can really travel, and that sambas, jitterbugs and even polkas all come under the ballroom umbrella. Ballroom dancing can be a real fitness workout.

Charles Lusch, M.D., oncologist and director of oncology services at Reading (Pennsylvania) Hospital and Medical Center, has been dancing for ten years, ever since he had a heart attack and seven bypasses.

"My health problems had forced me to give up my favorite hobby—race-car driving. Ballroom dancing filled the gap," he says. "I still jog and play tennis, but I defy most joggers to do three minutes of the samba and not be a little breathless.

"The variety of the workout makes it hard to be bored, and it's also easy on the musculoskeletal system. My wife suffers from osteoarthritis, and she feels distinctly better when we've been dancing regularly. People tend to see dance as a workout for the legs, but the upper body is very important, too. I think it's a more complete form of exercise than jogging."

Dr. Lusch recommends dancing to many of his patients, particularly women who've had breast cancer.

"Dancing is really adaptable. You can start out with simple, slow steps, and gradually work up to a vigorous workout," he says. "It's a great stress reducer. It's hard to keep your mind on your problems when you're swirling around the dance floor. And it helps to create a positive body image. My breast cancer patients say it restores their sense of femininity."

Phil Martin, dance teacher and lecturer at California State University at Long Beach, put ballroom dancing to an aerobics test. He and Betty Griffith, Ph.D., a physical-education specialist, tested a group of students with one semester of social dance and found that 62 percent could reach their target heart rates long enough to produce a conditioning effect on their hearts. And unlike some activities, where the more proficient you become, the more difficult it is to get your heart really pumping, experienced dancers have an easier time reaching aerobic levels.

Martin and Dr. Griffith took six intermediate dancers (with two semesters of training) ranging in age from 26 to 73 and put them through a routine of cha-cha, swing, polka, samba and Viennese waltz. All were able to attain and maintain their target heart rates for the 20 minutes necessary to gain a conditioning effect.

Thomas Allison, Ph.D., of the Mayo Clinic's Cardiovascular Health Clinic, says dancing can burn as many calories as walking, swimming or riding a bicycle. He says half an hour of moderate, sustained dancing can burn between 200 and 400 calories.

For the Health of It

Which is not to say that you have to swing and sweat to get any benefit from taking to the dance floor. Many of the health bonuses can be found far below the aerobic conditioning levels formerly recommended, according to John Duncan, Ph.D., associate director of the Department of Exercise Physiology at the Kenneth Cooper Aerobics Research Center.

In a study conducted at the center, two groups of women walked regularly—one at a normal pace, the other at a brisk pace. The brisk-pace group (walking a 10-minute mile) increased the efficiency of their hearts; the normal-pace group (walking a 20-minute mile) showed a slighter increase. But both groups raised their HDL cholesterol levels and lowered their total cholesterol, reducing their risk of developing coronary heart disease.

"The fitter person can do more work and have more endurance and stamina," says Dr. Duncan. "But we now know that moderately fit people can have hearts as healthy as superfit people. While being very fit can bestow certain physical benefits, we need to separate fitness from health. Regular participation in ballroom dancing certainly confers health benefits. How fit you become depends on how vigorously you dance."

A Real Crowd Pleaser

The new interest in ballroom dance crosses generations. The over-60 crowd dances cheek to cheek from memory. And baby boomers and their offspring—who grew up with freestyle, partnerless pumping on the dance floor—learn the joys of moving in sync with another human being.

"My evening classes have a wide variety of ages," says Martin. "The 'kids' learn from the older people and vice versa. It's really nice to see that kind of interchange. And my college students go home and dance with their parents and see them in a whole different light. I remember one girl coming back from vacation after going dancing with her father and saying, 'He seemed like a different person. I saw a side of him I never knew existed.' Take away the traditional roles and human beings show through."

Robert Black is state director for Pennsylvania's United States Amateur Ballroom Dance Association (USABDA), a national nonprofit network of 9,000 social dancers and amateur competitors that promotes ballroom dancing. He agrees it's a great way to get to know people. When his wife died of lung cancer, he plunged into deep depression. He coped by staying at home, sitting in his room and writing. His sister encouraged him to go out dancing, and "it changed my life," he says.

"I joined USABDA because I felt dance had really given me something, and I wanted to give something back." And that's just what he did. In less than 18 months he created so many new chapters that the state of Pennsylvania now leads the nation in number of chapters.

"While ballroom dancing seems to have attracted the over-50 age group, that's changing," he says. "One USABDA chapter president is 26. When you meet people dancing they don't want to know how old you are. They want to know how well you dance!"

Sociable Cross-Training

Dinner's over, it's dark and cold outside. You didn't get your walk in today, and your mind is thinking "exercise bike," but your spirit is shouting "Boring!" What's a body to do? How about putting on some lively music and inviting your spouse to take a spin around the living room?

Many people appreciate finding an exercise activity they can do with their spouse or friend. Not only does dancing avoid the isolation of solitary workouts, it may even coax unwilling exercisers into activity. It just looks like fun, not work!

Dr. Lusch admits that finding an activity he and his wife could enjoy together was a real plus for ballroom dancing. "We're both busy people," he says. "It was great to find a fun way to exercise together."

Bob Meyer, East Coast editor for *Amateur Dancer,* the national publication of USABDA, feels sorry for his jogger friends. "They're out there in the heat and cold, with the bugs and the sunburn and smog," he says. "I'm in a beautiful, temperature-controlled room with a graceful woman in my arms. And I'm getting the same benefits.

"My doctor always knows when I'm getting ready for an amateur competition and really dancing a lot. My resting pulse drops from 72 to 60! And I love that 'dancer's high' when you travel around the dance floor with another person in perfect balance, as one unit. That's joy!"

Stress Reducer and Positive Mood Builder

"Dance is a thinking person's sport," says Phil Martin. "You have to concentrate to be good. That helps keep your mind off other things. Learning new steps can be great for your sense of mastery and self-esteem. I've seen a number of students with poor grades begin to get As and Bs after they started at my dance classes. Dancing brings them out socially and gives them a sense of confidence."

Andy Orochena divides his concentration between flying 737s for USAir and twirling his dance partner, practicing for amateur competitions. Andy used to run but finds dancing "much more fun." "I sit a lot on my job," he says. "Dancing gives me an enjoyable physical and social outlet and helps me keep my weight down. Flying around the country can make it hard to regulate your food choices."

Andy loves competing and puts in as much as 15 hours a week of practice time. "It doesn't drain me, it rejuvenates me," he says.

Getting Started

Once you become interested in dancing, you may be amazed to find out how much is going on right in your own backyard. Aside from the famous franchises like Arthur Murray and Fred Astaire studios, which sell a kind of elegance as well as dance lessons, you can check out local Ys, local recreation bureaus, community colleges and independent studios for group lessons. They can be as low as five dollars an hour with a two- or three-hour practice session afterward. Often you don't need a partner, so singles needn't be discouraged.

"In our classes at California State, we change partners every few minutes," says Martin. "People seem to learn more quickly and are able to dance with anyone, not just one partner. Some couples resist at first, but when they see how helpful it can be, they join in the group."

If you're a bit shy about trying to master something new in a group, you may want to take private lessons or rent or buy dance videos. With videos you can rerun instructional segments over and over till you get it right. And

How 30 Minutes of Exercise Can Save Your Fat Budget

As we explained in Chapter 2, a person who exercises can eat more grams of fat a day than a person who is inactive. In fact, for every 100 calories you burn during exercise, you can eat three more grams of fat. In the accompanying table, we've taken 15 common exercise activities and calculated the number of grams of fat you can add to your personal fat goal if you engage in that activity for 30 minutes. We've included two common body weights, 130 and 170 pounds. If your weight is between 130 and 170 pounds, you can easily estimate an "Additional Grams of Fat" number.

Activity	Additional Grams of Fat	
	130 lb.	170 lb.
Aerobic dancing (medium)	5	7
Ballroom dancing	3	4
Basketball	7	10
Bicycling (leisurely)	5	7
Digging in garden	7	9
Golf	5	6
Jumping rope (moderate)	9	11
Ping-Pong	4	5
Racquetball	9	12
Running: 15-minute mile	7	9
9-minute mile	10	13
Swimming: fast crawl	8	11
slow crawl	7	9
Tennis	6	8
Universal gym	6	8
Volleyball	3	4
Walking	4	6

you don't have to have a partner to learn your part. After you feel comfortable, ask someone to join you or look for a group lesson.

Check your local newspaper. It may list USABDA chapter dances or nightclubs (which are beginning to offer free group lessons as part of the evening's entertainment). USABDA chapter dances always have an hour of instruction before the dance begins, so be sure to arrive on time. The more you dance, the more you'll find out about places to dance.

Dance clubs are also starting to flourish. They hold members-only dances and are for more experienced social dancers. Some even require an audition for membership.

What you wear can vary from place to place. Ask when you call, or find out from people who've been there before. One poor fellow in a suit showed up at a swing dance to find everyone "gettin' down" in shorts and T-shirts. The next night he went to a ballroom dance in jeans and a short-sleeved shirt and left when he found the women in sequins and the men in jackets and ties. At country-western nights, cowboy boots and ten-gallon hats may be de rigueur.

While competition dancers still prefer high heels on women, Martin suggests flats. "Heels shorten the tendons in the back of the leg, put too much stress on the ball of the foot and pitch your weight forward," he says. "We encourage flexible, flat shoes for dancing." Sometimes even sneakers work. It depends on the dance floor. Too much traction and you stick and squeak. Too little and you slip and slide. Again, ask around and learn by trial and error.

But don't wait for an evening out to learn your steps. Practice at home, either alone or with a partner. Find your favorite music and waltz around the living room. Play a video and tango along. You may find that you dance at a lesson one night, go out for an evening of nightclub dancing and spend an evening or afternoon practicing at home.

That adds up to a whole lot of fun as well as a fair share of healthy exercise!

The Secret to Sticking with Exercise

The benefits of regular exercise have been widely publicized for years. So why do so few people exercise? And why do most of those who start an exercise program drop out after three to six months?

Over the years, researchers have blamed exercise dropout on everything from personality type to poor instruction. But you want to know the single most important step you can take to keep yourself exercising?

On every day that you planned to exercise, go out—at the same time—whether you exercise or not. If you planned on doing a circuit at the local gym, at least go over and watch others do it. If you were going to run for 45 minutes, at least go out and walk for 5.

Psychologists who have been studying exercise behavior for over a decade say you have to get into the habit of taking time out of your day for exercise. Just get comfortable with being there when you said you would.

Some research shows that flexible goals like these are extremely important in sticking with an exercise routine. Strict or overambitious goal deadlines that you impose on yourself can simply serve as reminders of failure. For more tips on how to stick with exercise, see Chapter 6.

CHAPTER

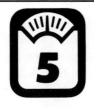

YOUR FEELINGS AND YOUR PHYSIQUE: THE MIND/BODY FACTOR

Everyone knows how to lose weight: You have to burn more calories than you consume. With some fine adjustments (we now favor moderate but consistent exercise like brisk walking over strenuous activities, and low-fat, as well as low-calorie, menus), the fundamental rule of weight loss hasn't changed in decades. Unfortunately, neither has our success in mastering it; only about 10 percent of those who manage to take off excess weight keep it off permanently.

It's not for lack of trying—or lack of programs to try. So, what's missing? According to our experts, the best pounds-off program is doomed if you're not mentally or emotionally prepared. To succeed, first you've got to tap the weight-loss power within your own head.

Psych Up to Slim Down

"The best plan for weight loss begins in the mind," says Thomas Wadden, Ph.D., director of the Center for Health and Behavior at Syracuse University. "Most people talk themselves out of losing weight. The challenge is to talk yourself into it." Here's how.

Think Small

"Permanent weight loss means making small, manageable changes and sticking with them for life," says Michael Hamilton, M.D., director of the Duke University Diet and Fitness Center.

Of course, change is never easy. It often feels threatening, especially when it's "for life." That's why it's important to decide which changes are small enough to feel manageable and nonthreatening. In other words, which changes are no big deal?

When Steve Purser, who's with the San Francisco public health department, felt ready to lose weight, he made only two changes: "I cut out alcohol, and instead of diving into sweets after dinner, I took a walk. If I still wanted dessert after my walk, I'd have it. But usually, when I got home, I felt fine going without it."

"Making drastic short-term changes never lasts," says fitness instructor Joan Price, author of *The Honest Truth about Losing Weight and Keeping It Off.* "To keep weight off, make small changes over time and incorporate them into your life. Make lifestyle changes at your own pace," she adds.

When pondering possible changes, Trish Ratto, a registered dietitian and associate director of health promotion at the University of California at Berkeley, advises, "Be honest with yourself. Don't even consider a change you're unwilling to stick to. If you can't live with it, it won't become permanent."

How should you make your changes? First, list all the little things you're truly willing to do. Maybe you can't give up frozen desserts, but it's no sacrifice to switch from ice cream to frozen yogurt. Perhaps you're repulsed by jogging, but it's no big deal to park one block farther from the mall and walk the extra distance. Or maybe you can't live without burgers, but you're willing to switch from cheeseburgers to plain hamburgers. These changes may sound insignificant, but they're not.

Let's say you normally drink about two glasses of milk per day and decide that you can make the small change from whole milk to skim. That small change will save you about 463 grams of fat a month—or about 1 pound! That's 12 pounds a year!

"It's the small changes that become permanent," Ronette L. Kolotkin, Ph.D., director of behavioral programs at the Duke University Diet and Fitness Center, says, "and permanence is crucial. I applaud switching from cheeseburgers to hamburgers—if it's for life."

Once you've listed all the changes you can live with, rank them from easiest to hardest. Then make your easiest change—and no other. As soon as it becomes a permanent habit, make change number two and so on. "When you no longer have to struggle with one change," Price says, "it's no big deal to make the next."

Here's a small, realistic goal: Begin by holding the line for six months; that is, don't try to lose weight, just maintain your present weight. "That's a real success," says Dr. Wadden. "It can provide confidence that helps you move on to actual weight loss."

Take a Mental "Breather"

Once you've made the decision—and commitment—to change, pick a starting date in the not-too-distant future. Give yourself a couple of weeks to ponder your decision and psych yourself for success. Don't just dive in. When Steve Purser made his decision to lose weight, he knew he was prepared to forgo alcohol and substitute walks for desserts—but he didn't plunge right in. "I waited until the first of the year. I'm not really sure why. It just felt right."

For some people to ensure a successful outcome, they need to choose a start date that's personally meaningful: their birthday, a child's birthday or perhaps the anniversary of some event that pushed them to make the commitment (for example, the date of an overweight relative's heart attack). So they don't lose momentum, the start date should not be more than a month from the day of commitment.

Be Realistic and Patient

"It's simply not realistic to want to lose 50 pounds in two months," Dr. Wadden says. "A realistic goal is 5 pounds in two months."

"For permanent weight control, losing a half pound to a pound a week is plenty," Dr. Kolotkin explains. "Tabloid headlines like: 'Lose 15 Pounds in a Week' train people to be terribly impatient about weight loss. Quick fixes never

work. Weight doesn't come off quickly. If you're not ready
to give it time, you're not ready to lose."

Enjoy Physical Fun

No one loses weight permanently by diet changes
alone. "The problem," Joan Price explains, "is that it's very
difficult for longtime couch potatoes to get off the sofa."
Her solution? "Don't call it 'exercise.' Start by becoming a
little more physically active in your daily life."

Price, 48, speaks from experience. An uncoordinated
child, she hated gym and didn't learn how to swim or ride
a bike until her midtwenties. "The only physical activity I
liked was dancing—I had no idea it was 'exercise.' "

"Exercise" doesn't mean sweating buckets doing
things you hate. That attitude keeps couch potatoes in
Spudville. "Half of those who start exercise programs stop
within a few months," Price explains, "and half of those
who stop do so before their first session. Many give up in
advance because they try to force themselves to do things
they don't enjoy."

To find something you like, Price suggests recalling
the activities you enjoyed when you were younger—basket-
ball, Ping-Pong, tap dancing, whatever. Take one up again,
or try something close. Price's girlhood love of dancing led
her to aerobics. "Find what works for you," she says.

Price seconds fitness authorities who recommend
three or four half-hour workouts a week. "But not immediately," she insists. "That activity level should be your ultimate goal. If you're getting ready to become more physically active, a half hour can feel intimidating. To start, try
going just five minutes a couple times a day. That can
change the experience," she says.

"Instead of feeling defeated before you start, you'll feel
positive. Five minutes? You can do that." Soon five becomes
ten, and when you're ready, you can last an entire class.

Don't Expect Perfection

"Most people expect themselves to be perfect," says Arizona weight-loss psychologist Susan Olson, Ph.D. "They're so hard on themselves. When I ask how they view themselves, they say: 'I'm a refrigerator with a head' or 'a balloon with legs.' Preparing to lose weight means realizing that everyone makes mistakes. Forgive yourself."

Consider marriage. When spouses fight, they don't immediately get divorced. After most marital mistakes, spouses forgive each other. That's part of any permanent relationship. Permanent weight control is similar. It means entering into a new, more forgiving relationship with yourself. You are starting over. "We're only human," Ratto explains. "I use the 80–20 rule. I watch what I eat 80 percent of the time. The other 20 percent, I don't worry about it."

The quest for perfection leads to preoccupations with two other weight-loss demons—willpower and guilt. "Dieters misunderstand the cause of being overweight," says Jean Antonello, R.N., author of *How to Become Naturally Thin by Eating More*. "It used to be believed they ate too much and had no willpower and should feel guilty for being 'bad.' Of course, it's got nothing to do with guilt or willpower. Dieters have willpower but are starving, and no matter how much willpower they muster, after a while they lose control and binge. This is because their bodies' survival instincts take effect. But when people eat quality food whenever they get hungry, appetite normalizes and the body asks for less food."

Yo-yo dieters are often so disgusted with themselves that they become incapable of even recognizing their accomplishments, let alone celebrating them. "If they lose weight, they credit the diet," Dr. Olson says. "If they don't, they blame themselves."

If you have trouble seeing how far you've come, create some charts, not just of your weight but also of the number of minutes you walk each day or the flights of stairs you climb. Or take pictures of yourself on the first of each month and post them.

Part of cheering your progress involves rewarding yourself, not with hot fudge sundaes but with other treats. "Even after one week of walking 30 minutes a day, treat yourself to a new pair of walking shoes," Price suggests, "or to a weekend at a health spa after six months."

Plan to pace your rewards so that you earn at least one a week. "Don't fall into the trap of saying, 'I'll do this or that after I've lost 30 pounds,'" Dr. Wadden says. "To lose weight permanently, you have to become your own cheer-leader. Don't lament, 'I only lost half a pound this week.' Say, 'All right! Another half pound! That makes seven pounds in ten weeks. I'm doing it.'" In other words, be your own cheerleader and someday you might look like one.

How to Eat Wisely under Stress
By George L. Blackburn, M.D., Ph.D.

Associate professor of surgery at Harvard Medical School and chief of the Nutrition/Metabolism Laboratory with the Cancer Research Institute at New England Deaconess Hospital, Boston

All of us know that there's a relationship between the amount of stress we feel and the way we eat. Some of us clam up under pressure: We can hardly swallow a bite. Others of us soothe ourselves from morning till night with "comfort" foods, like cookies, ice cream or chocolate. Poor choices, in turn, compound fatigue, anxiety and weight problems.

Unfortunately, this tactic leads to more stress and more weight problems.

Here are some positive nutritional guidelines to follow to help break the stress cycle.

◆

1. Drink water. Water is the most overlooked essential nutrient. When the going gets rough, many people experience dry mouth, sweating and heart palpitations. They're all caused by a stress-induced imbalance in the sympathetic nervous system. Also, many people who stop eating under stress also forget to drink liquids, which can lead to dehydration and more severe symptoms. Drinking plenty of water in stressful times rebalances the system, prevents dehydration, counteracts dry mouth and heart palpitations, and replenishes fluids lost by sweating.

2. Eat fiber. Stress often goes right to the gut, where it can cause cramps and constipation. Fiber counteracts these problems. Build up to 30 grams of fiber a day by gradually adding more fruits, vegetables and whole grains. Breakfast is a major fiber opportunity: Eat whole fruits (instead of just juice), enjoy whole-grain cereals and fiber-fortified breads and muffins.

3. Don't skip meals. Stress has many components, like anxiety, depression and fatigue. Skipping meals accentuates those problems. A breakfast rich in carbohydrate, protein and fiber is particularly important. The morning meal stimulates the sympathetic nervous system; it revs up hormones and neurotransmitters in the brain for an active day. If a person goes without a healthy breakfast and lunch, it's much more difficult to concentrate or get work done—making the day's tasks even harder.

4. Focus on variety. It's better to try to eat a lot of different foods, rather than try to get specific nutrients. Scientists just don't know enough yet about nutrient needs to say, "If you're facing a deadline at work, you'll need more of vitamin X, Y and Z." So include nutrient-rich foods from the four food groups (grains, low-fat dairy foods, lean meats and fruits and vegetables). The proper attitude: "Okay, maybe I can't avoid these deadlines at my job, but I don't have to trash my body by eating junk food."

5. When ill, think nutrition. On the other hand, under the stress of an illness, people may need extra amounts of specific nutrients, particularly water. In case of a serious cold that kills the appetite, added amounts of vitamins B, C and E from a multivitamin can be beneficial. (If you have a more serious illness, talk to a physician or nutritionist about an eating plan that incorporates extra amounts of easily digested, nutrient-dense foods.)

6. If overeating under stress is a problem, pay attention! The first thing to do is to recognize the new, unhealthy eating pattern. Keeping a food record in a small notebook is a good idea. Consume healthy snacks—100 calories per serving—and drink plenty of water. Become a grazer rather than an eater of large meals. Then make a conscious effort to override the bad habits by filling up with healthy foods and engaging in moderate physical activity to reset the appetite to normal. (See number 8 below.)

If you're scarfing down meals too quickly, try to become aware of every mouthful. Cut and chew each bite slowly, savoring the flavor, and sip water frequently while keeping your attention focused on the food. You'll appreciate the food more—and probably eat less.

7. If stress ruins your appetite, it's okay to eat less. At least for a few days. A 50 percent reduction in food, or "modified fasting," is okay for three to five days, especially if you remember to drink plenty of fluids. One solution is to drink a "meal replacement" shake like a commercial liquid breakfast to help meet nutrient requirements. In the meantime, exercise to rebalance and stimulate your appetite and to improve digestion. If the fasting continues longer than a few days, consult a physician or nutritionist.

8. Exercise moderately. Believe it or not, exercise can both quell and stimulate the appetite—depending on what's needed. For people eating in an uncontrolled way, moderate exercise increases metabolism, reduces stress and seems to aid in appetite control.

If the appetite is meager, moderate exercise like walking can stimulate gastric secretions and aid digestion, to make us more receptive to food. The key is moderation. Stay in tune with your body.

9. If stress brings sleepless nights, back off the coffee and caffeine-containing tea. Caffeine-containing drinks, of course, can make it harder to fall asleep and stay asleep. Give up caffeine for a few days and see if your sleep and mood improve. The inability to sleep deeply and wake feeling rested is a sensitive index to major stress, particularly if it's recurrent. Your physician can help you assess whether your problem requires medical attention.

10. Say no to sugary snacks. Sugary snacks taken independently of a meal—like an afternoon candy bar— can send some people on a blood sugar roller coaster. They may provide a quick jolt, followed by deeper tiredness and anxiety. I'm talking specifically about sugared snacks with no nutrients or fiber in them, such as many carbonated beverages and sugary drinks. On the other hand, if you take your sugar in moderation as part of a meal, it won't trigger the highs and lows. Choose fruits and milk-based products, like low-fat frozen treats, for dessert.

11. Incorporate nutrition into the big picture. Remember, you can't separate nutrition from other health habits that combat stress. While a modest degree of stress is part of a busy lifestyle, disabling stress that deprives you of sleep and stamina needs special attention. Exercise, as we've pointed out, encourages healthy eating. Getting enough sleep, managing time efficiently, maintaining a sense of humor, meditating and dealing constructively with stressful situations all contribute to healthy nutrition—and they're all important pieces of an antistress program.

Turn Off Your TV and Turn On Your Weight Loss

"Warning: Excessive TV watching can lead to obesity, high cholesterol, disturbed intellectual function and negative emotional states. Keep watching at your own peril."

Is it possible that you may be seeing a warning along those lines flashed on your TV screen every half hour in the not-so-distant future? We think it is, even if you are the one mentally flashing that message to yourself after each program. Because it's true. But even better would be a message saying: "GOOD NEWS! By turning off your TV, you may well cut your risks of becoming overweight, or staying overweight, in half. In addition, this step may help you lower your cholesterol, concentrate better, feel better, communicate more with your family and friends, and generally get a lot more out of life." Because that's true, too.

Most of us already realize that unchecked "tube-o-philia" is less stimulating and satisfying to the brain than about 500 other activities.

What is most disturbing is the link between TV and weight. The more you watch of the first, says increasing evidence, the more you will have to watch the second.

The unhealthy relationship begins when daily viewing time reaches three to four hours a day, explains Larry A. Tucker, Ph.D., professor and director of health promotion at Brigham Young University in Provo, Utah.

In one study, Dr. Tucker and colleague Glenn M. Friedman, M.D., studied over 6,000 working men whose average age was 40. They discovered that those who spent more than three to four hours a day watching television had twice the risk of being obese as men who watched less than one hour. Obesity was defined as having 20 percent to 30 percent body fat. Chances of being what they call super-obese—31 percent or more body fat—were more than doubled.

Dr. Tucker and Marilyn Bagwell, R.N., Ph.D., reported similar findings in the *American Journal of Public Health*. Studying a population of nearly 5,000 working women, average age 35, they discovered almost the same fattening trend.

Again they found three to four or more hours of total daily TV watching to be the point at which the chance of being obese doubled. The interesting thing about four hours is that it's the typical amount of time an American spends watching TV each day. So the average person, male or female, is just at the point where they have doubled the risk of becoming not only a couch potato but a stuffed couch potato.

Tube fixation is, in fact, second only to working for a living when it comes to gobbling up the hours we spend on waking activities. And for children, watching TV is their primary waking activity—the only thing they do more of is sleep. On a global basis, it's been estimated that the people of the world spend over three billion hours watching TV each day.

Wheel of Misfortune

All this doesn't establish a definite cause-and-effect relationship between heavy TV watching and heavy people. "But there is a definite link or interaction," says Dr. Tucker.

"I believe much of the problem is cyclical," he suggests. "As television viewing time increases, physical activity time decreases. As physical activity declines, fitness also tends to decline. And as fitness declines, attraction to passive recreation, such as TV viewing, increases."

It's cyclical, all right. Just like "Wheel of Fortune." But the only prize some people win is 25 extra pounds of fat they don't really want.

The connection between TV viewing and fading fitness has also been documented by Dr. Tucker. In a study published in *Research Quarterly for Exercise and Sport,* he compared TV viewing time and fitness levels of almost 9,000 adults. People who watched for less than one hour a day were the most fit. Compared to them, viewers with a three- to four-hour habit were 41 percent less fit, and those who did regular four-hour-plus marathons of viewing were 50 percent less fit. Right about now, Jack LaLanne is gnashing his teeth.

Are Tucker's findings exaggerated, perhaps? No way. A study of nearly 800 adults published in the *Journal of the American Dietetic Association* found that, while the incidence of obesity among those watching an hour or less of TV a day was 4.5 percent, prevalence shot up to 19.2 percent for those watching four or more hours a day. Here, the risk didn't double—it quadrupled!

That study also found the apparent fattening effect of TV is not just a result of failing to get exercise. Feasting on TV seems to produce fat all by itself. Even if you get some exercise, in other words, watching lots of TV is so sedentary that the good effect of exercise can be diminished.

Nor is it just a matter of people gorging on goodies while they're tube-tied. Putting aside the effect of extra snacking they may do in front of the TV, heavy viewers are still putting on the poundage at an accelerated rate.

And, if already obese, they are much less likely to overcome the problem. Curiously, the average consumption of calories seems to have gone down over the last 10 to 20 years, yet both teenagers and adults are heavier than ever. During that same period, though, TV viewing has been documented to have increased by about an hour a day per person. And that's not counting all the time we spend watching movies on the VCR.

In any weight-loss program, then, adjustments in TV viewing habits may have to be made if you really want to succeed, suggest authors Steven L. Gortmaker, Ph.D., and colleagues from the Harvard School of Public Health and Tufts New England Medical Center.

The Cholesterol Channel

Obesity, of course, is a known risk factor for a number of all-too-common health problems, including diabetes, high blood pressure and high cholesterol—all of which can translate into heart disease. But TV excess has been linked with elevated cholesterol in a fairly immediate way, even in kids.

In one study, researchers found that children who watched two or more hours a day of TV had double the chance of having high cholesterol as those who watched less. Kids who watched for four or more hours a day had four times the risk.

"Aside from not getting any exercise," says Kurt V. Gold, M.D., "when you sit and watch TV, you're not only exposed to more fast-food and junk-food advertising but you may also tend to snack on these foods you're watching. This tendency may contribute to the higher cholesterol levels associated with excessive TV viewing."

Dr. Gold, who worked in conjunction with the American Academy of Pediatrics on the research, tells us that he and his colleagues tried repeatedly to disprove the TV/cholesterol link. But they couldn't. "At the present time," says the physician, now at Loma Linda University Medical Center in California, "overexposure to television is a greater predictor of high cholesterol in children than anything else we have looked at."

Whether the same TV/cholesterol link exists in adults is currently under investigation, Dr. Gold says.

Emote Control

Of course, no one expects a session of TV watching to make them healthier. But many believe it is a good way to relax and shed the cares of a tough day.

Well, cancel that thought. A study supported by the National Institutes of Mental Health and conducted on 1,200 subjects over 13 years concluded that watching television for long periods of time leaves people in worse moods than they were in before they began to watch. In fact, when people sit down to watch TV specifically to escape their troubles or feel better, the exact opposite occurs. In addition, the more TV people view, the less able they are to concentrate overall.

These mood and cognitive changes may be more than minor. "Personally," says Dr. Gold, "common sense tells me that TV addiction can contribute to depression. The images that television puts before us, that we have to look and live like Tom Selleck's or Cybill Shepherd's characters do, can be depressing and can undermine self-esteem. That's especially true if your lifestyle and appearance are a lot different from those portrayed on television," he adds.

Irritability, difficulty relating to others and boredom may also be linked to excessive television viewing. It seems the more TV viewed, the worse off you may be in terms of your positive mental state. In *Television and the Quality of Life: How Viewing Shapes Everyday Experiences,* by Dr. Robert Kubey and Dr. Mihaly Csikszentmihalyi, a compilation of studies spanning 13 years, researchers reported that reduced social interactions and negative moods are linked to heavier television viewing. It was found that, among the sampling of divorced and separated subjects, levels of irritability increased dramatically with the increased amount of TV watching. Other researchers found that twice as much television viewing was done by clinically depressed adolescents than was done by a control group of "normal" teenagers.

◆

"Perhaps the most devastating thing about TV viewing is that while you're watching television, you are less likely to accomplish anything else," says Dr. Gold. "As an audio-visual, TV engages much of the viewer's brain but very little of the body otherwise. The result is tremendous energy drain without the benefits of healthy physical activity."

Some would say you aren't just inactive physically but intellectually and emotionally as well. In this sense, excessive TV becomes a wedge between your consciousness and your life, focusing all your attention on only the superficial, artificial and irrelevant.

Are you concerned about your TV watching habits? Worried that your favorite program is becoming your diet downfall? Here's a list of the shows considered "most addictive" by many doctors and specialists: soap operas, sporting events, high-action shows and situation comedies.

Are You a Victim of TV?

Put a check mark next to each question you answer with a "yes."

1. Do you watch more than two hours a day of television?

2. Do you cease to communicate with others while you are viewing TV?

3. Do you become unhappy or irritated after you must turn the television off to do something else?

4. Do you, from time to time, feel extremely tired during a regular day's schedule?

5. Do you frequently eat junk food or unhealthy snack food when you sit down to watch television?

6. Do you experience frequent insomnia and use TV as a means of distraction during your sleeplessness?

7. On a pleasant day, are you more likely to stay indoors and watch television than go do something outside?

8. Is it difficult for you to share and communicate your feelings and experiences with others?

9. Are you actively involved in less than two hobbies, clubs or sports at least four hours a week?

10. Do you frequently turn on the television and search the stations without having a specific program in mind to watch?

Grading Yourself

For every odd-numbered question you answered yes to, give yourself two points. These factors were determined by our experts to be indicators of too much television watching. For every even-numbered question you answered yes to, give yourself one point. These factors, in conjunction with poor viewing habits, signal possible trouble. Tally your score, then use the following scale as a rating guide.

3 or less points: No problem
4 to 6 points: Potential trouble brewing
7 to 9 points: Excessive television viewing
10 points or more: Eek! Your brain is becoming fused
     to your TV's circuitry. See "The TV Detox Program."

The TV Detox Program

There's no need to throw your television in the trash to cure a severe case of TV-aholism. "One remedy would be to wean yourself off TV," says Alan Caruba, founder of the Boring Institute in New Jersey (a popular media spoof, which also looks at the serious aspects of boredom). Take the TV section of your Sunday paper and mark off all the programs you really want to watch. Then stick to the schedule! Turn on the set only when the shows you selected the previous Sunday are on and be sure to turn the TV off when those shows are over.

And, remember, no flicking through to other stations; that habit leads to mindless viewing.

When the TV is off, Caruba suggests the recovering TV addict get out of the house. Go outside and do some gardening, walking, visiting friends, anything but sitting around. If you don't leave the house, leave the room where a television is tempting you to turn it on. Read something, write a letter, pick up an old hobby or start a new one. Replace the inactivity of TV viewing with an activity that you like.

Kurt V. Gold, M.D., a physician at Loma Linda University Medical Center, agrees with Caruba's preselection method. "Spend more time thinking about what you are doing. That's how to gain control of any drug or medication, and that's how to gain control of your viewing," says Dr. Gold.

"It depends on the type of television viewing, as well. There are educational programs that are not the big culprits involved with mindless TV time. Unfortunately, the more popular programs are not necessarily documentaries or news programs," says Nathan Wong, Ph.D., assistant professor in the Department of Medicine at the University of California Medical School at Irvine.

Slow Down and Slim Down

Do you have more work, more weight and more stress than a body should bear?

Join the crowd. There's a raging epidemic of "too much to do and never enough time to do it"; "working hard and worrying about work"; "free time? what free time?"; "if I'm not under tremendous stress I must be dead"; and "how the heck did I get on this roller coaster?"

To cope, some people lash out in all directions at once, always starting but never finishing anything. Others procrastinate, so today is always spilling over into tomorrow, and they're always late. Many, already burdened past endurance, choose to make their lives impossible by taking on more.

Something has to give and usually does—quality time with your family gets scarce, your health suffers, weight control is out of control.

It's the Overweight-Overwhelmed-Overworked syndrome. What to do? Beat the O's. Most of us can't stop working, but we can work smarter. We can't shirk responsibilities, but we can set saner priorities. We can't avoid stress, but we can adopt strategies that minimize it. We can't expect to be at the perfect weight all the time, but we can avoid the self-defeating cycle of weight gain that all too often accompanies stress.

Here are four realistic ways to do it.

Take a Walk

Regular walking is one strategy that can attack all three O's at once. It can help you lose weight; give you the perfect opportunity to sort out goals, priorities and schedules; and reduce stress in a big way.

A number of studies over the last several years have supported the use of exercise as a natural stress reducer. One of the more recent involves police officers, who know a thing or two about stress and overwork. Those who undertook a ten-week program of aerobic exercise showed marked improvements in physical health, as well as their perceived sense of stress.

Another report on correctional officers showed similar good results. By the conclusion of a 6½-week workplace exercise and wellness program, most of the prison guards had lost weight, lowered their cholesterol, increased their muscular endurance and showed a higher tolerance for stress.

But wait. How can an overworked, overweight, overwhelmed person find the time for regular walks in the first place? Well, research suggests that regular exercise like walking can make time. It can increase your stamina and energy, which can enable you to get more done in less time. So investing 20 to 30 minutes a day in walking may actually save you more time than that.

Just Say No

"Stressed-out people often can't assert themselves," says Joan Lerner, Ph.D., a counseling psychologist in private practice in Philadelphia and a psychologist at the University of Pennsylvania Counseling Service. "And so they swallow things. Instead of saying, 'I don't want to do this,' or 'I need some help,' they do it all themselves. Then they have even more to do."

Asking for help seems obvious, but for many it's not. Instead, many overwhelmed people keep their resentment—and their work load—all to themselves, explains Sally Ann Greer, Ph.D., a Virginia psychologist who specializes in stress management and weight reduction. Asking for help and learning how to say no are skills that the overworked must practice.

"You can teach people how to say no tactfully," says Merrill Douglass, president of the Time Management Center in Marietta, Georgia, and coauthor with his wife, Donna Douglass, of *Manage Your Time, Manage Your Work, Manage Yourself.* Often, saying no at work is a matter of giving your supervisor choices, Douglass says. "Say, 'I'd really like to take this on, but I can't do that without giving up something else,' " he suggests. " 'Which of these things would you like me to do?' " Most bosses can take the hint, Douglass says.

Also, he suggests, examine your reasons for not saying no. Some people don't say no because it makes them feel guilty. "They don't say no because it might create a conflict," he says. "But often the people who keep asking you to do more don't see it as a conflict. It becomes a vicious circle, and you have to slow it down."

Get Your Signals Straight

Overwork often triggers stress. But instead of finding a way to reduce their anxiety, some people respond inappropriately, often seeking solace—or maybe just distraction—by eating.

"Food is a comfort. On an unconscious level, I believe people who are stressed get their signals confused," says Dr. Greer. "They begin to interpret stress as a signal to eat rather than as a signal to reduce stress in their lives."

Some people, of course, eat less when they're stressed out. Others eat more. Whether you eat more may have something to do with whether you're overweight in the first place.

A number of studies suggest that overweight people eat more food in response to stress. A more recent report, however, suggests that if you're overweight to begin with you may use food as a constant mood elevator, even when you're not under stress. So-called normal-weight people, in contrast, tend to eat less when under stress and eat more when they've had a good day. Those who tend to eat when overworked need to pay more attention to what they're feeling. Stress signals not the need for bonbons but for rest or relaxation.

When you feel the urge to eat, ask yourself if you're really hungry. If you aren't, Dr. Lerner recommends exploring what she calls nonedible alternatives. One of the women she counseled in a weight- and stress-reduction program at the University of Pennsylvania would go out on her break and buy a single red rose instead of a snack. "There are other ways to fill yourself up," she says. In a national study, "The Mitchum Report on Stress in the '90s," for example, 75 percent of those polled said that they listened to music to help alleviate stress.

Still other people use food not as a way to cope with stress per se but as a means of avoiding dealing with the very thing that's driving them crazy in the first place.

"Food is kind of like a diversion," explains Dori Winchell, Ph.D., a psychologist in Encinitas, California, who specializes in eating disorders. "It's a way for you not to fix what needs to be fixed. You hate your job and you hate your boss, so you are miserable. You say, 'I might as well be nice to myself. I might as well eat some ice cream.' "

The more appropriate response to those signals of distress is to confront what's really making you fed up. Easier said than done, Dr. Winchell acknowledges. But she adds, "If you are living the life you want to be living, I guarantee stress is not going to make you overeat."

Other options, according to Paul J. Rosch, M.D., president of the American Institute of Stress: "Try progressive muscular relaxation. Alternately tense and relax the muscles of your body, going from one group to the next, shoulders to arms to hands, and so on. Other people use visual imagery or meditate."

And if you must eat, try low-fat alternatives like seasoned, unbuttered popcorn or nonfat frozen yogurt.

Put Time on Your Side

Stressed-out people often seem overworked because they're simply disorganized. If a project is due Friday, they start working feverishly on Thursday. Either that or they apply themselves with equal vigor to every task, even though some tasks are more important than others. So they feel out of control—a leading cause of workplace anxiety, according to time-management consultant Merrill Douglass.

If you recognize the symptoms of disorganization in your work habits, Douglass recommends the following steps:

Use a notebook. Make a list of your responsibilities and check them off as you go along. Most pressing tasks go at the top, and the least time-sensitive go toward the bottom.

If you're not a list maker, try a scan-card system.
Sold in stationery stores, these are folders that open up to
reveal a number of pockets or slots, each of which contains
a little card. Write each responsibility on a card, and put it
back into a slot. As you complete a task, throw away the
corresponding card. A variation on this theme, which
Douglass also recommends, is to write your daily chores
on yellow Post-It notes, and throw each one away as you
finish the task written on it. In this way, you can see progress, and you can see what remains to be done.

Whatever system you use, Douglass notes, it ought to
be compatible with your work style. "If it adds too much
structure to your life, you're unlikely to use it," he says.
"Time-management techniques have to be compatible with
who you are and how you're going to use them."

Set deadlines for yourself. These are important because they aren't imposed by others. Without self-imposed
deadlines your work may expand to fit your time and probably tempt you to put everything off.

Set long-term goals. "Most people don't have any
goals," says Douglass. "But people who have goals, who
are actively pursuing them, probably feel in control of most
things and also feel less stressed. They may be working just
as hard, but they feel that they're getting somewhere. The
feeling of stress has less to do with your work load than
with whether you're in control of your workload."

Delegate. Overworked people often get that way because they believe they have to do everything themselves.
They don't. Organized, efficient people have mastered the
art of sharing tasks or delegating them to others, including
family members.

Winter Weight Gain May Be Linked to Seasonal Blahs

People suffering from seasonal affective disorder, or SAD, are more likely to gain weight during the winter months, and as many as 15 percent of patients being treated for obesity have SAD, according to obesity specialist and Medifast physician Fred Yates, M.D.

Dr. Yates is director of the Center for Nutrition and Weight Management in Seattle and is a member of the American Society of Bariatric Physicians, a group dedicated to the study of obesity.

SAD is a form of depression that has been linked to lack of sunlight and is particularly pronounced in regions of the country where daylight differences between summer and winter are significant. SAD is also cumulative. Its most severe effects are felt in late March and early April, when suicide rates soar and the number of people seeking help for depression reaches a peak. One of its symptoms is increased appetite and weight gain.

"It's normal to gain three or four pounds this time of year," Dr. Yates says. "All mammals become less active in the winter. We hibernate, and stay inside because the weather is overcast and the days are short, and become less active as a result. Studies show the less active we are, the more our appetites are stimulated, so we eat more. For the person with SAD or a severe case of the winter blahs, however, the weight gain can be as much as 30 to 40 pounds."

Couple this natural tendency to overeat in the winter with SAD, and a recipe for obesity is born. For those already obese, SAD saps the energy necessary to start exercise programs or take other steps to lose weight.

"One in five obese patients experiences seasonal bouts of depression and weight gain," Dr. Yates says. "Often, we find if we treat for one medical condition, we affect the other. For example, obese patients who start diet and exercise programs find their SAD is mitigated. Likewise for patients being treated for SAD. As the depression lifts, they find they have more energy to tackle weight problems."

SAD is reported predominantly in women between the ages of 20 and 45. No one knows why this particular group appears to be affected more than others, but some researchers hypothesize it is because younger women visit physicians more often, are more likely to seek medical help for weight problems, and are less disposed than older groups to accept seasonal depression as normal or unimportant.

To be diagnosed with SAD, at least three of the following clinical symptoms have to be present: depression, lethargy or lack of energy, sleep disturbance or increased appetite and weight gain. Luckily, there is treatment.

"Phototherapy is a rapid and effective treatment for winter depression. This involves sitting under a high-intensity, very white light that filters out ultraviolet rays and simulates natural sunlight. In one study, patients who sat under the light for at least 30 minutes a day experienced a 75 percent remission rate. This same study found the most effective time for phototherapy was early in the morning." Dr. Yates says.

Dr. Yates cautions, however, that only patients with a clinical diagnosis of SAD should undergo phototherapy. "SAD mimics other depressive illnesses. Phototherapy could have disastrous effects on patients who are manic-depressive, for example," he says. "The light actually can induce mania. It's important that if you suspect you have SAD, you see a doctor."

For milder cases of the winter blues, Dr. Yates offers the following tips:

• Get outside as much as possible, especially in the early morning hours, to maximize exposure to sunlight.

◆

• Exercise, exercise and exercise. "Exercise makes you feel better. It burns calories and increases your production of endorphins, a pleasure-producing hormone manufactured by the body. Exercise suppresses appetite, and also makes your body work more efficiently," Dr. Yates says.
• If all else fails, plan a winter vacation where the sun is shining.

"Excessive weight gain and depression are not inevitable by-products of the winter season," Dr. Yates explains. "There is no reason to suffer. SAD can be treated. Your family physician is your best source for information on obesity and seasonal depression."

Stressed Out? Hit the Road

Webster's Dictionary defines stress as "that which strains or deforms." Put too much stress on a piece of metal and it breaks. Put too much stress on your body or mind and it begins to suffer the consequences: fatigue, tension and anxiety, illness.

When we're under stress, our body releases chemicals that, although helpful in the short run, become harmful in excess. Walking helps you to dissipate those harmful chemicals immediately. And walking regularly helps to condition you so that stressful events take less of a toll. A regular walking program, then, is a great stress buster.

But there's another way to bring the beneficial effects of walking to bear in your life. Instead of just using walking to wash away the effects of stress and protect against its onslaught, there are many times when you can take a walk to avoid stressful situations altogether!

Here's a list of seven stress-busting walking strategies:

1. Feed your feet, not your face. If anxiety, boredom or force of habit have you running to the refrigerator for comfort, slow down! You're just making life more stressful by adding excess weight. When you know your hunger is motivated by stress, force yourself to take a brisk walk around the block or the hallways instead. Walking can relax you and may help you lose the urge to eat under duress.

2. Relieve "eyeball" pressure. Take your spouse, your boss, your child or your friends for a walk-and-talk session. Meeting with people face-to-face, where constant eye contact is required, can generate extra anxiety and tension, especially if the subject matter is stress-producing to begin with. Whenever you can, plan walking encounters. Not only do you relieve stress by making continual eye-to-eye contact unnecessary, you both get to walk off some of the tension as you talk.

3. Take walk breaks at work. Escape from the office routine of coffee and doughnuts. Research shows that a brisk walk can give you more energy than eating a sugary snack does. If you can get outside, the fresh air may do wonders for your outlook, too. If not, a brisk jaunt through the halls, and maybe a flight of stairs, can bring you back to your desk ready to concentrate.

4. Park in your driveway. Ever head downtown on a Saturday morning and spend precious time circling the stores looking for a parking space? Try leaving your car at home and walking to town for your Saturday morning errands. You can avoid the aggravation of clogged streets, not add to the local pollution and benefit from a relaxing stroll. You may even save time!

5. Incubate afoot. Sometimes knotty problems can leave us feeling physically tied in knots. That's the time when less thinking and more relaxing and mental drifting can be a real asset. Take a stress-free stroll and let your subconscious do a little undercover work. Leave the problem behind, and when you get back, you may just find the answer staring you in the face.

6. Avoid parking-lot panic. Door dings, kids everywhere, cars pulling in and out. Parking lots sometimes seem like accidents waiting to happen. Next time you head for a mall or department store, don't automatically head for the center of the storm and try to get the choice spot closest to the door. Park as far from other cars and the entrance as you can. Take a stroll around the perimeter before you race into that bustling shopping arena. A restorative cooldown will be waiting for you on the way back to the car.

7. Plan a walking vacation. Vacations are a sign of status in America. Everybody wants to take one. But we do it so seldom we're not very good at it. Planning a vacation can be a big headache. All the details, the reservations, the restaurants. How many people come home saying they need a vacation to recuperate from their vacation? A walking vacation, on the other hand, is a truly rejuvenating experience. Tour companies around the country are cropping up that literally take care of your every need for a weekend, a week or more, at destinations here and abroad. You eat fine foods, walk through beautiful, scenic pathways and meet wonderful people. And all you have to worry about is the daypack on your back. You come home invigorated and refreshed. And looking forward to a walking vacation can add incentive to your walking program.

Ask your travel agent for brochures on walking tours. Or join the *Prevention* Walking Club and receive discounts with tour companies we've already tried and loved. For more information write to: *Prevention* Magazine Walking Club, 33 East Minor Street, Emmaus, PA 18098.

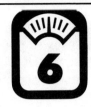

THE 93 BEST WEIGHT-LOSS TIPS OF 1993

There's no way around it. Losing weight is a challenge. And anyone who has tried to drop those extra pounds knows that sometimes the going gets really rough. That's why we interviewed the experts and spoke with dozens of people who have successfully shed extra pounds, looking for the best tips to help make the going a little easier for you.

Why be modest about what we've found?

These are absolutely the best tips of the year. True, these tips debunk a few myths, but maybe those myths need debunking. By the time you've browsed all 93, you'll be on track for '93. Not only that, you'll notice that some things you've heard about weight loss and exercise just aren't true. And some things you can do to give your weight loss plan a big boost are easier than you thought.

Basic Pointers for Trimming Down to Size

1. Develop a healthy nutrition plan. Studies show that people who diet without a well-structured plan struggle harder to lose the weight. It's important to put some clear principles from Chapter 1 down in writing. Think of them as your long-range goals for healthier eating. Post them on the refrigerator door or right over the kitchen counter so you can periodically remind yourself.

2. Make a schedule. Write down a time frame for accomplishing specific parts of your diet goals. For example, within a month, phase out the use of butter. Or, within two months say: "I'll *never* eat when I'm depressed!"

3. Remember the five-hour rule. If you go five hours without eating, you will very likely become so hungry that you no longer care about weight loss. If you eat something before five hours, you maintain a sense of control over food choices. Result? *You,* not *your hunger,* have the control.

4. Carve out a healthy pattern. Keep a food diary and identify your eating patterns. What time of day do you eat? What mood are you in when you eat? If necessary, revise these patterns so that you consume breakfast, lunch and dinner at regular intervals.

5. Establish a fat budget. Check the table on page 21 to see how many grams of fat you should be eating per day. Begin to look at the fat content of the foods you eat. Modify some of those choices so you select lower-fat foods whenever you can.

6. Resign from the clean plate club. So many people clean their plates today because of old messages they received as children. We end up eating twice what we really need. Examine your need to clean your plate by asking yourself, "Am I still hungry?" when you've half finished the food on your plate. And if you're not, guess what? You *don't* have to finish.

7. Sip instead of snack. As you go through your day, try to keep a cup of water nearby and take occasional sips. It not only helps you meet your body's need for water and gives you a sense of fullness, it may also prevent food cravings.

8. Brush away cravings. Before giving in to that craving for a piece of candy, try brushing your teeth. The sweetness of the toothpaste may take your craving away, and with the flavor it leaves in your mouth, who needs a handful of jelly beans?

9. Abstain from alcohol. In one study, researchers found that people who had more than two drinks a day had much larger waist-to-hip ratios (potbellies) than nondrinkers. In fact, the drinkers were bigger all over than the nondrinkers.

10. Stop puffing. In the same study, researchers found twice as many fat abdomens among smokers as

◆

nonsmokers. Several other studies point the finger at smoking, too. So if you haven't given up smoking yet, now's the time. (P.S. Quitting, contrary to popular myth, *won't* make you fat.)

11. Start huffing. Research continues to show us that exercise is an important way to achieve long-term success in a lose-weight strategy. But many people find it difficult to work exercise into an already packed schedule. If you are serious about losing weight and keeping it off, you may have to reorganize your schedule. Treat yourself to an exercise program—*any* exercise program. A daily walk, for instance, is an excellent way to start. Do just enough today so you look forward to doing it again tomorrow!

12. Lose it once. Weight is more dangerous the second (and third) time around. Scientists have found that people who lose and regain weight repeatedly tend to carry a higher percentage of body fat. That means every time you lose and regain weight, you regain *more* weight than you did the time before. The following tips will help you avoid "weight cycling."

Attitude Adjustments That Make Slimming Easier

13. Rethink your ideal. Wanting to look good, and be reasonably trim, is a sensible goal. But wanting to look like a fashion model isn't. Recognize the basic body shape that you have inherited. Accept this shape and feed it a healthy diet to achieve good health, not a stick figure.

14. Spend some time on yourself. While you're working on your body, it's important to keep your self-esteem in good shape, too. Buy yourself a few flattering clothes, try a new hairstyle or take time to do little things that make you feel special. Positive self-esteem will help power you through your weight loss.

15. Accept yourself. This can be tricky and may take a little practice, but you absolutely must learn to accept yourself the way you are before you can lose weight. Many people do the opposite and make self-acceptance contingent on weight loss. By doing that, they are adding so much tension and stress to their lives that they end up turning to food for relief. If you learn to like yourself first, you'll treat yourself better, and weight loss will follow.

16. Demystify the "bad" guys. There is no doubt about it: A carrot is a healthier snack than a piece of candy. But snacks are only small components of your overall diet. Within the framework of a daily diet, there is room for almost anything—in small amounts. The problem with categorizing all foods as either good or bad is that it gives them a kind of power they really don't deserve, and then you want them more. Don't punish yourself more if you slip and indulge in a piece of candy. A peppermint piece now and then *doesn't* have the power to scuttle your diet plan.

17. Be sure you are ready. Before you begin a weight-loss program, make sure you are extremely motivated with your goals very clear in your mind.

18. Remember you're in it for life. Make sure that you are committed to maintaining a healthy diet and increased exercise for life. Remember this is not a "diet" that you will start and end at specific times. It's a new, healthy way of eating and exercising that will last your whole life and ensure weight loss.

19. Start at the right time. Don't start a weight-loss program under difficult life circumstances that you feel may jeopardize your chances for success. Just about to make a big move? Having major problems with a spouse or significant other? These are *not* the times to launch a weight-loss program.

Foodwise Tips for Healthy Weight Loss

20. Boost your intake of produce and grains.
The long-standing basic "four food groups" recommendation was two servings a day of fruits, two servings of vegetables and four servings of grains (bread and pasta, for example). Now we're on to something better, especially for weight loss: The 1990 Dietary Guidelines have increased the recommended numbers to two fruits, three vegetables and six grains every day. These food groups are high in complex carbohydrates, fiber and many vitamins and minerals. Slowly try to incorporate more vegetables, including dry beans and peas, into your diet. And eat more fruits, breads, cereals, pasta and rice rather than dairy products, meat and fats.

21. Keep the Twinkies out of your kitchen. What you buy at the grocery store and bring into your kitchen is what you will most likely end up eating. Even if you really bought Twinkies "just for the kids," guess who might get to them *before* the kids. The time you spend at the food market is a crucial time for your whole weekly diet. What you buy is what you eat. Don't shop when you're feeling hungry. Wait until you're in the right frame of mind to make these important choices for the week.

22. Know your "-ose's." Read food labels for clues on sugar content. If sugar, sucrose, glucose, maltose, dextrose, lactose, fructose, corn syrup or any other syrup appears at or near the top of the list, there is a large amount of sugar in that product. Look for "-ose"-free products instead.

23. Be careful of your combinations. Americans love to combine simple sugars and fats in the same meal—a hamburger, french fries and a cola, for example. When the body gets a jolt of simple sugars, as from a soda, it releases lots of insulin in response. Insulin is a storage-prone hormone, which "opens up" fat cells, preparing them for fat storage. Add the fat from the burger and fries and it's bad news for your hips. The idea is to go on a low-fat diet, and when you do consume fat, don't consume simple sugars with it.

24. Reject "fad" diets. Stick with a sensible diet that relies on fruit, vegetables and other low-fat fare, and emphasize slow, gradual weight loss. Don't fall for any of the many bizarre diets out there. They are bound for failure.

Mealtime Nuggets . . . of Weight-Loss Wisdom

Here are a few quick and easy tips, specially designed to help you eat light at mealtimes.

Breakfast

25. Get flaky. Start your morning with a heaping bowl of cereal and you'll likely eat less fat and cholesterol throughout the day—even compared to those who eat something else for breakfast, according to research at St. Joseph's University. High-fiber cereals that contain at least 4 grams of fiber per serving are the best choices, but you can find an ever increasing variety of low- or no-fat cereals.

26. Measure up. While you're pouring out your cereal, check the nutritional information on the box for fat content. But beware: Most cereal boxes list very skimpy servings as the average serving size. You'll probably have to multiply everything by two if you want to find out what you actually pour in the bowl. And that means doubling the fat content, too.

27. Move toward margarine. Although margarine has about the same fat content as butter, it's lower in saturated fat, and that's the really bad kind of fat. Go for the "low-fat" or "light" versions of margarine now available.

28. Soften up. Warm margarine to room temperature. Softer bread spread means using less. Chances are, you'll end up with one-quarter of the fat and calories if you put it down at room temperature rather than cold. If you forget, use the microwave.

29. Best of all, spread on the fruit. To spurn fat entirely, spread your toast or bagel with fruit preserves or jam, which are fat free, instead of margarine. You'll save about 4 grams of fat for every pat you don't use.

30. Slim with skim. Although whole milk contains only 3.3 percent fat, that measurement is by weight. The true, meaningful measurement of fat is actually percentage of calories from fat, and 49 percent of the calories in whole milk come from fat. "Low-fat," or "2 percent," milk isn't much better: Fully 35 percent of its calories come from saturated fat. But skim milk gets only 5 percent of its calories from fat.

31. Redo your brew. In coffee, a little low-fat milk makes a decent substitute for half-and-half, with less fat. Better yet, use evaporated canned skim milk, which has no fat at all.

32. If you just can't eat breakfast, drink it. Some people just can't face food in the morning. If you're one of them, a good quality liquid instant breakfast is better than nothing. Look for a product that's low in fat and sugar and that provides a third of the Recommended Daily Allowances of vitamins and minerals.

Lunch

33. Try a new twist on tuna. Here's a low-fat version of tuna salad. Combine a can of drained, water-packed tuna with a tablespoon of red wine vinegar and chopped onions to taste.

34. Make a healthy lunch mix. Turn a can of low-sodium broth (beef or chicken) into a quick, healthy meal by adding fresh or frozen vegetables, cooked chicken chunks or diced tofu, fresh or dried herbs and a little freshly grated ginger and/or hot pepper sauce. To defat the broth, refrigerate it for a few hours, then skim off all the fat that congeals on the top.

35. Detour around the deli. Deli sandwiches with all the trimmings can be loaded with trouble. Stay clear of the fatty sauces and avoid salt- and smoke-cured meats like bologna, ham and salami. However, without sauce, turkey or even lean roast beef sandwiches are fine.

36. Bag it. No matter how you slice it, going out for lunch every day is a fattening proposition. It's much easier to control your diet and eat low-fat fare when you pack it yourself. See our tips on packing healthy lunches on pages 88 to 96.

37. Miss the mayo. Try some fancy mustards or even horseradish on your sandwich. They add a more flavorful perk to your sandwich than regular mayonnaise at almost no cost to your fat budget.

Salad Bar Savvy

Salad bars can provide the fixings for a nutritious, filling and low-calorie lunch—or a fat-laden dietary disaster. Here's how to make smart choices.

38. When it comes to greens, branch out! Ignore the iceberg lettuce in favor of spinach, romaine or leaf lettuce. They contain more vitamin A and calcium.

39. Load up on the right stuff. Dip deep into the beans, peas, beets, sliced mushrooms, cucumbers, tomatoes, green pepper, grated carrots, broccoli and cauliflower. Go for the freshest-looking vegetables. The ones in sauces and dressings may be thinly disguised fat carriers.

40. Eat like a mouse. That is, the amount of cheese a mouse would eat. Grated cheese is almost always included at salad bars, but it adds a lot of unnecessary fat to your otherwise lean lunch.

41. Favor fish and fowl. If you want a garnish of meat, pick the shrimp, chicken or turkey. Only 20 percent of their calories come from fat.

42. Eliminate the extras. Skip the ham, chopped eggs, croutons, bacon bits and fried noodles and the salads made with mayonnaise.

43. Go barely dressed. Use no more than one tablespoon of dressing, even if reduced-calorie is available. (The round dippers on most salad bars are the equivalent of two tablespoons.)

Dinner

44. Pick a perfect prelude. Start with a high-carbohydrate food, like a pasta appetizer, bread without butter or a bean or noodle soup. That will lessen your appetite.

45. Learn a new chicken trick. Oven-fried chicken tastes great—without a trace of added fat. Rub skinless chicken pieces with prepared mustard, then coat them with yellow cornmeal. Bake at 450°F for 15 minutes, then lower the temperature to 350° and bake another 20 minutes, or until cooked through.

46. Feel fuller with fish. In a new study of food and fullness, people who ate fish dinners felt more satisfied and full than people who ate either beef or chicken. And after the meal, the feeling of fullness lasted longer for the fish-eating group than for the other two. That's useful news for people who get hungry and pig out between dinner and bedtime.

47. Love seafood—but skimp on shrimp. Seafood is good food, low in saturated fat and rich in artery-protecting omega-3's. And shellfish lovers should take note that clams, mussels, oysters and crabs, once suspected of harboring too much cholesterol, have now been cleared of artery-threat charges. But shrimp delivers surprisingly high amounts of cholesterol. Steer clear.

48. Get to the meat of the matter. We have no beef with beef, as long as it's eaten in moderation. To make sure you get the leanest meat, check the grade. "Prime" and "choice" cuts are the highest in cholesterol. What makes them so tender and juicy is fat. The "good" and "select" cuts have less fat, fewer calories and less cholesterol.

49. Rack 'em up. Grill your steaks or cook them on a rack or slotted pan to let some of the remaining fat drip away. Never rub a steak with oil before cooking it; that will seal in most of the fat.

50. Perk up your potato. You can make a baked potato flavorful with a few drops of extra virgin olive oil, soy sauce, horseradish or Worcestershire sauce or an herb-and-spice blend. Or try this topping: Mash tofu with a little low-fat mayonnaise, then add curry and herb seasonings to taste. (Or just a tablespoon of low-fat yogurt might do the trick.)

51. Try a "garden variety" pizza. Make your own pizza dough (or buy it ready-made), but instead of the usual toppings, try vegetables like carrots, onions, fresh tomatoes, peppers and broccoli. These toppings can either be stir-fried in a tiny bit of oil or, better yet, steamed. Top with part-skim mozzarella and bake as usual. Instead of pepperoni, sprinkle on some ground turkey or turkey sausage that you've taken out of its casing.

Dessert

52. Nuke a fruit. For a fast, nutritious, low-calorie dessert, microwave an apple. First peel the top third to prevent the insides from bursting as the heat expands them. Cover the apple and cook on full power for three minutes. Top with yogurt flavored with half a teaspoon of maple syrup and a dash of cinnamon.

53. Try the perfect parfait. Here's another low-fat dessert. Put a layer of diet Jell-O in a tall glass, then a layer of low-fat vanilla yogurt, another layer of Jell-O, one more of yogurt and top the parfait with fresh strawberries.

Snacks

54. Select your freezer snacks. A frozen juice bar (almost no fat) is a much more healthful cool snack option than an ice cream bar (15 to 25 grams of fat). If you *must*

◆

have something cold and creamy, go for a pudding pop (about 2 grams of fat).

55. Dish it out. Never eat foods out of their original containers. It's easy to lose track of what you're eating. Your intentions may be "just to taste" but pretty soon you're "finishing off" that pint of ice cream. You're likely to eat much less if you dish out the food in a measured portion and put the container back in the refrigerator.

56. Monitor your munchies. Choose pretzels over potato chips. Pretzels contain about 1 gram of fat per ounce; many chips have ten times that much. Plain, air-popped popcorn is a good snack choice, too.

57. Add an apple. An apple is not only a great low-fat snack, it may also keep the dieter's droopiness away. Scientists at the federal government's Human Nutrition Research Center in Grand Forks, North Dakota, found that boron-rich foods improve motor skills and boost alertness. Apples and other noncitrus foods such as broccoli, peas, beans and cabbage are good sources of boron, which also helps the body retain calcium.

58. If you must eat cookies . . . keep in mind that, in general, the more the cookie crumbles, the better it is for you. Softer-textured cookies tend to have a higher fat content. (One of the exceptions is fig bars.) Harder cookies like gingersnaps and vanilla wafers have about half the fat of their soft cousins.

Recipe Renovations That Cut Half the Fat

Here are a few handy substitutions you can make to cut the fat from your favorite recipes. You'll be surprised how good everything tastes even when low-fat replacements step in!

59. Spray it on. If your recipe calls for sautéing vegetables in oil, use a no-stick spray or a flavored liquid, such as defatted chicken stock or vegetable juice. Some vegetables with a high moisture content, like onions and mushrooms, can create their own liquid, so you don't need any other sautéing liquid at all. Cover tightly in a nonstick pan on low heat, stirring every few minutes. When they've given off enough of their own juices, you can add other foods to be sautéed.

60. Ditch the cream. When your recipe calls for heavy cream to thicken a soup, use buttermilk or evaporated skim milk instead. Many "creamed" vegetable soups can get along without the dairy thickener altogether. Just scoop out about a cup of cooked vegetables, whir in your blender and return to the pot for creamy thickness.

61. Give meat a head start. When cooking meat and vegetables together in a stew, simmer the meat with seasonings a day ahead, then refrigerate the stock overnight. The following day, remove the fat that has congealed on the surface of the stock, add the vegetables and cook until they are tender.

62. Amend your milk. When recipes call for milk, use nonfat or skim milk; just to be sure add one tablespoon of nonfat dry milk per cup as a thickener.

63. Taste this tasty cake. Lots of recipes for cakes and muffins call for vegetable oil. Try replacing the oil with applesauce. You'll get a moist, naturally sweet result.

64. Try an egg-cellent trick. Substitute two egg whites for every egg that your recipe requires. Egg whites are completely fat free and work well in place of whole eggs.

65. Move to a higher ground. When recipes—lasagna, for example—call for ground beef, use ground turkey breast (no skin) instead.

How to Stick with an Exercise Program

66. Lay out your exercise clothes the night before. Sometimes seeing them there the next day helps remind and inspire you. It also eliminates part of the "getting dressed" hassle.

67. Dress casually. Wear exercise clothes around the house and town (so you'll be ready when the urge strikes). Sometimes how you're dressed influences how you feel. In this case, you may feel more like exercising.

68. Have equipment, will exercise. Always carry exercise equipment in the car (again, so you'll be ready).

69. Rub elbows with fitness fellows. Spend time with others who exercise. Their habits really will rub off on you. You may even like to exercise together.

70. Skip the bar hopping. If you want to exercise after work, avoid drinking buddies and bars at that time. Sure, there's peer pressure! Just turn it around. Instead of going out for a drink, invite your peers to go exercise.

71. At least *get there*. Drive to the gym at the appointed time, even if you don't feel like exercising. Once you're there you might as well get into exercise clothes. And after that . . . well, why not work out?

72. Solicit support. Tell your friends to keep asking you about your exercise. The encouragement and support will help you along. It's always good to have a friend you can share your successes with.

73. Surround yourself. Put up signs, pictures or posters that remind you of exercising. Positive images go a long way.

74. Expand your aerobic repertoire. The more activities you enjoy, the more you are likely to do all around. Take up *anything* just for the novelty of it. Try walking, roller-skating, volleyball, tap dancing—the possibilities are endless. In fact, don't call it "exercise." Call it "fun." Having fun is the best revenge against exercise dropout.

Recharge Your Routine

75. Calculate your workout. To figure out how hard you should be exercising, follow this simple formula for target heart rate zone. Subtract your age from 220. The number you get is the factor for the next two steps. First, multiply the number by 0.60 and then go back and multiply the number by 0.80. The two numbers you get will be your target heart rate zone. When you exercise your heartbeats per minute should be in that zone.

For example, if you are 40 years old, you would subtract 40 from 220. Then multiply 180 by 0.60 (108 beats a minute would be the low end of your goal). Then multiply the 180 by 0.80 (144 beats per minute would be the high end of your heart rate goal).

While you are exercising, periodically check your pulse to see if it's within your range. (You can count your heartbeats for ten seconds and multiply by six to get your heartbeats per minute.)

76. Stand up straight and let go. Let go of those bars on the side of the stair-climbing machine. Studies have shown that if you hang on to the sides of the machine when it's set at a level-12 workout, you're only getting the benefits of a level-6 workout. When the machine displays how many calories you've burned at the end, you can cut that number in half if you've been hanging on.

77. Check your biking posture, too. Same thing with exercise bikes. If you're hanging over the front of the bike, you're cutting the benefits of the workout by a good 30 percent. Sit up straight on the bike; you'll get more out of it, even if the RPMs are lower.

78. Easy does it with the weights. Lifting faster won't make you stronger. It's intensity, not speed, that activates those fibers. You want to raise the weight with a nice, even stroke and then bring it down slowly. If you let momentum shove it up and gravity drop it back down, you're defeating the purpose.

79. Fit in fitness. If you're more than 30 percent above your ideal weight, exercising before a meal will burn up more calories. If you're less than 30 percent overweight, exercising after eating burns more calories. (To avoid indigestion, however, you probably won't want to do any serious aerobic exercise too soon after eating a heavy meal.)

80. Externalize. Pay attention to what's going on around you, not inside you. Some research suggests that highly trained athletes do better when they pay attention to their bodily sensations. But for those who are just beginning to exercise, it's the worst possible strategy. Outside distractions help take your mind off the aches and pains. But do pay attention to pain and dizziness or a light-headed feeling—your body may be telling you that you're overdoing it.

81. Give yourself an A for effort. Be generous in evaluating your performance. Even if all you did was show up, pat yourself on the back for not skipping out. There will be plenty of time later on to compete against yourself or peers . . . after your exercise program has been firmly established.

Unmasking Common Myths about Exercise

82. Sweat loss is not fat loss. Many people weigh themselves before and after a workout and say, "Wow! I lost half a pound!" But what they lost was water, and they'll put it back on again the first time they have a drink and rehydrate themselves. Sweat loss doesn't equal fat loss—in fact, some studies say that excessive sweating is a sign that you're going too fast to burn fat.

83. Not all aerobics classes burn fat. In a 30- or 40-minute aerobics class, you spend 10 minutes warming up, 10 minutes cooling down and 10 or 15 minutes lying down doing floor exercises. You're only moving aerobically for 10 or 15 minutes. And you need at least 20 minutes of continuous movement to start burning fat. It's true that shorter classes will help tone you up, and they're certainly better than sitting at home. But the shorter classes won't burn fat like a half-hour on a ski machine or a treadmill.

84. You won't burn much fat on a "timed" workout. A lot of computerized exercise machines, like the StairMaster and the Lifecycle, have preset, preprogrammed, 15-minute workouts. They benefit your heart, but you have go for at least 20 minutes to burn fat. Program it yourself instead, or do two programs in a row without stopping in between. Go slow for half an hour and watch the fat start to fade away.

85. Sorry, sit-ups don't flatten your belly. They'll tone your stomach muscles, but they won't do much to reduce fat that covers those muscles. You can't spot reduce with exercise; if you could, people who chew gum a lot would all have thin faces.

86. Forget about the number on the scale. The scale is not a good measure of how well your exercise program is working. If you lift weights, for example, you'll lose flab; but because you're losing fat tissue and replacing it with denser, heavier muscle tissue, your weight may stay the same. The important thing is, you'll look better, feel better and fit into your clothes better, and you'll know it without even glancing at the scale.

87. Running won't ruin your cycle. If you're a woman who's running just to lose weight (and not competitively), you probably won't do any harm to your menstrual cycle. Researchers in Canada found that, contrary to popular belief, women could run up to 30 miles per week and still suffer no negative effects to their menstrual cycle.

88. When you stop, muscle doesn't turn to fat. Hard muscles may degenerate into soft muscles, but they won't turn into fat. Muscle cells and fat cells are completely different, and neither can ever turn into the other.

89. It's not dangerous. Many people avoid exercise because they're afraid of getting hurt. Actually, injuries are far from inevitable. In fact, the majority of exercisers don't get hurt. When they do, the most common cause is overuse. The best way to avoid injuries is to increase the intensity and duration of your exercise gradually.

90. Sweating doesn't mean you need extra salt. You'd have to shed three quarts of sweat to lose just a fraction of the salt you consume in a day. Since it's highly unlikely you'll sweat anything close to that amount, there's no reason to add extra salt to your diet or to take salt pills after hot weather workouts.

91. Don't wreck your neck. Despite popular opinion, sit-ups should not be done with hands behind your neck. It puts too much pressure on cervical vertebrae. Keep your hands on your chest, or lightly rest your fingertips behind your ears.

92. Hypertensives, you can lift weights. People with high blood pressure have often been advised not to lift weights. And it's true that if you have any cardiovascular problems, you should see your doctor before undertaking a strength-training exercise program. But long-term studies of weight lifting and blood pressure have failed to show any negative effects, and some have demonstrated that the exercises can reduce blood pressure.

93. It doesn't have to hurt. The "no pain, no gain" slogan is a thing of the past. You can get very fit without feeling any serious discomfort, so don't strain when you train. If something hurts, stop doing it.

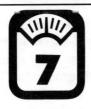

SPOTLIGHT ON THE SUPERCHAMPS: REAL-LIFE BODY MAKEOVERS

Need a little inspiration? Nothing like a true-life story about someone who fought the battle of the bulge and won! All the people in this chapter have one thing in common: They turned their lives around with exactly the kind of weight-loss plan you're reading about in this book. Meet the real-life success stories—and read how they did it.

She Lost Over 100 Pounds and a Big Pain in the Back

Nancy Myers of Parkersburg, West Virginia, was at a crossroads in her life. On the verge of turning 40, the 5 feet, 2 inches crossing guard had reached a milestone with her weight—240 pounds. And her back was feeling the brunt of it. With her cholesterol creeping upward, too, she believed if she didn't slim down soon, she'd never do it. So she stepped into action. Nancy moved from life on the sidelines to life in the fast lane, and bypassed her usual fare for leaner cuisine. The result? She dropped 105 pounds! And six years later, she hasn't turned back.

"I had always heard it was almost impossible to lose weight after 40. And at 39 I was 240 pounds.

"I had been heavy all my life. When I was young, I had tried to lose weight all the wrong ways. I took diet pills. I took laxatives. I made myself throw up. When you're a teenager without any dates and you think it's because you're too fat (I weighed as much as 170 pounds), you'll try anything to lose weight.

"Sometimes I lost weight, only to regain it, and then some. But as I got older, I gained more steadily. When I got married and had my first daughter, I gained 50 pounds; with my second daughter, I gained even more.

"I wasn't active at all, and my eating habits were pretty poor. I could sit down at night and eat four or five peanut-butter-and-jelly or bologna sandwiches. I loved all kinds of

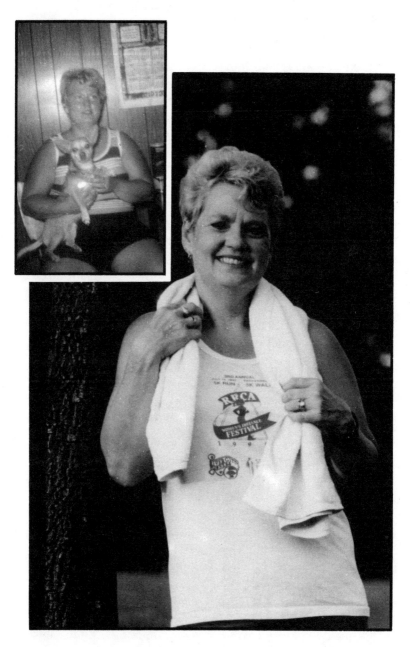

Walking—then running—Nancy Myers left 105 pounds in the dust!
She also got rid of her lower back pain, her high blood pressure and
her high cholesterol.

fattening sweets like cakes and pies. I thought, 'I'll drink diet soda to balance out the calories.'

"I didn't care how much I gained. But when my daughters got a little older, I started working as a crossing guard at a grade school. And then people I didn't even know started making fun of me. Strangers would holler things like, 'Don't walk on the sidewalk! You're gonna crack it!'

"I acted like it didn't affect me, but it did. And my weight was starting to affect my health, too. I had such severe muscle spasms in my lower back—worsened by my weight—that I had to be taken to a hospital several times. Though my blood pressure was in a safe range at 120/80, my cholesterol was definitely high at 233 [200 is the recommended maximum].

"But the turning point came the day before Valentine's Day 1985, when I walked up the stairs at my home and could hardly breathe. I decided that was it—it was time to try to lose weight for good. The following day, I gave all of my Valentine candy away."

Out of the Frying Pan

"I started by cutting out all the fattening sweets I used to eat—the candies, cakes and pies—and cutting out salt. I used to pour salt on every bite of food I took. But I knew from reading about health that salt makes you retain water and can raise blood pressure in people who are sensitive to it.

"I started eating three balanced meals a day—cereal with fruit for breakfast, a salad for lunch and a chicken or fish dish for dinner. I cut red meat out of my diet and I cut out lots of other fats. I'd never used a lot of butter, but I started using low-fat salad dressings rather than rich ones. And I started cooking differently. I used to fry everything, so I switched to broiling or microwaving, adding no fat whatsoever.

"I still loved sandwiches, but I stopped eating the fatty meats and started buying reduced-calorie bread. I ate tuna sandwiches without mayonnaise, topped instead with lettuce and tomato. In fact, I found I loved to eat plain tomato sandwiches!

"For snacks I ate celery, bananas or apples, and every once in a while, artificially sweetened candies to satisfy my sweet tooth. I also drank plenty of low-fat milk, which held me over between meals.

"But I knew dieting alone wouldn't help me keep off weight—I had tried that plenty of times. So I started to exercise, too."

Support on the Home Front

"My husband had had a weight problem until the year before I started my diet. Then he had started jogging and lost 65 pounds. I had never gone jogging with him because I was afraid of hurting my bad back—and I thought I was too fat. But when I started my diet, he suggested that I try walking. That I knew I could handle.

"I started out walking two to three miles twice a day between my shifts as a crossing guard. Then I'd walk again in the evenings with my daughter, who's very active and who encouraged me in my new activity. I started out slowly, figuring it would be difficult for me to breathe. But I found I could do it, no problem!

"Soon I started speeding up and increasing distance. After several weeks, I was walking five miles three times a day, every day except Sunday. The more I walked, the more I enjoyed walking! And after a few months of walking and eating right, the pounds just melted off. Instead of making fun of me, people were stopping to compliment me! By June I'd lost 80 pounds.

"But that same month my weight loss reached a standstill. And since I was still determined to lose more weight, I decided to join my husband and try jogging.

"I still felt fat, and I didn't want anyone to see me, so I went to a nearby cemetery that's two miles around. At first, I could only jog down the hills; I walked the rest. My breathing was very uncomfortable. But slowly I built up my endurance and I got used to breathing correctly. Soon I could jog the whole two miles!

"It took about three weeks to get me off my weight-loss plateau. Then I started dropping weight again. Over the next three months, I lost 25 more pounds! I also ran a two-mile race with some hills that, to me, seemed like mountains. I didn't place, but I did finish, and that was my goal.

"I loved jogging so much that I joined a runners' club. I started running races, and even won a few trophies in my age division. I've built up to running a nine-minute mile!"

Working Incognito

"By the time I reached my fortieth birthday that August, I weighed about 120 pounds. I had a big celebration—but without a cake!

"That fall, I got down under 120 pounds, but I felt I was too skinny. So I started eating a little more of the right foods—like skinless chicken, salads and fruits. I even allotted myself some sweets, like low-calorie cake. That way, I built my weight back up to 135, where I looked much better.

"All my work paid off. At 40, I was a different woman. When school started in the fall and I returned to my post as the crossing guard, people didn't even recognize me. The mailman who'd passed me for four years didn't know who I was!

"Now, six years later, my weight is holding at 135. My back problems are gone, my blood pressure dropped to 108/72 and my cholesterol is down to 200.

"I work in the evenings now, so I jog in the afternoons—four to eight miles a day. Instead of hearing nasty comments from strangers, I now get whistled at!

"I find that I can eat a lot more now and stay slim as long as I continue to eat a low-fat diet. I feel great about myself now. I'm never turning back!"

He's Funnier without the Fat

When he was a child, *John Passadino,* of Bellerose, New York, had learned that fat was funny. In school he'd clown around about his hefty shape to get his share of the spotlight. But at 29, the part-time actor and comedian realized his weight was no laughing matter. He had reached 212 pounds at only 5 feet, 7 inches. His cholesterol had climbed to 375, his legs cramped up and his breathing was labored. That was when he decided to get serious about weight loss. With a little self-education, he was able to write himself a new routine for living—with a sensible diet and exercise at center stage. And the results would make anyone smile.

"When I was growing up, people always said, 'He's eating, God bless him! He's healthy!'

"'Eat the fat,' they said. 'It'll keep you warm in the winter!' So I did eat the fat—and lots of it. I ate hamburgers, hot dogs, cakes and candy. It's no wonder I was the fat kid in the class. None of the girls were ever interested in me. That was why I became the class clown—to get attention.

"When I was in eighth grade, I weighed about 163 pounds and went on the first of many crash diets. I lost a lot of weight, but by high school, I'd put it all back on. After that I tried a lot of other crash diets—like a grapefruit or one-meal-a-day diet—to lose weight for special occasions, such as weddings. I'd lose about 20 pounds, but afterward my weight would go right back up.

"As I got older and began to moonlight as a comedian (I work full-time as a computer analyst), I used my jowly appearance to make me look funny. But all the while I feared the audience was just laughing at my body, not my jokes. I was afraid to lose weight—for fear of losing laughs.

"By June of 1988, my weight was causing major problems. I was experiencing muscle cramps in my legs. My breathing was so labored people could hear it when I talked to them on the phone. I'd reached 212 pounds and my cholesterol was 375.

"My doctor told me that I could develop diabetes as a result of my excess weight. And my elevated cholesterol was putting me at high risk for heart disease. My father had suffered his first angina attack in his late forties. I kept looking at all his medications and thinking, 'Am I going to have to do this when I'm in my forties? This is crazy! It's time to make a change.' And that's just what I did."

Learning a New Act

"I had never learned how to eat right, so I had to completely reeducate myself about nutrition.

"My first step was to get some books on health and nutrition from the library. I learned how much I should be eating to maintain my weight, and how much less I'd have to eat to lose some. I realized I would have to drastically cut my fat intake.

"I set out to lose about five to ten pounds. I cut out fatty red meats and opted for chicken without the skin. I stayed away from ice cream, and instead I ate more fruit. I made eggs my symbol of everything that was elevating my cholesterol and swore I would never eat another yolk.

"I also knew from my reading that I had to exercise if I wanted to lose weight and keep it off. But I had never been active in my life because my weight had turned me off to exercise.

"So I started out slowly. I began riding a stationary bike for just five minutes a day. It was so easy that each time I finished, I felt as if I hadn't done anything. But I knew

I would burn myself out if I did too much too soon. So I stuck with just a five-minute ride for two weeks.

"In the third week, I rode for 10 minutes a day. The following week, I rode for 15 minutes. I began losing weight very easily. I wasn't suffering from hunger pains at all.

"Within a month of my exercise program and fat cutback, I lost ten pounds!"

Rediscovering a Body

"After three months, I was riding for about 40 minutes a day. By that time, my cholesterol reading was down to 213! When I saw results, I really got into losing weight. I cut back my diet a little further. I started drinking low-fat milk instead of whole and eating low-fat yogurt and cheeses instead of the higher-fat versions. But I allowed myself pizza once a week for incentive. By January of 1989, I had stepped up my exercise program. I began weight lifting to tone my muscles, and I even started jogging. I started out slowly, jogging for just 15 minutes. Then I worked up to a half hour. Within six months, I was jogging for 40 minutes at a time.

"I was rediscovering my body, and it felt great to be able to do all the things I'd never been able to do in the past. I could play paddleball and ride my bike well. I didn't turn into an athlete, but I did feel more coordinated. And I never would have thought of jogging before I started my program!

"But then my joints started hurting. I had read that walking was as good as running, so I scrapped the jogging and took up walking instead. In addition to my regular walking regimen, I started taking the train to my comedy and acting jobs, getting off at an earlier stop and walking the rest. The walk was about 30 to 40 minutes each way, and I would take it two or three times a week. "By that spring I was down to 150 pounds, and my cholesterol was down to 196!"

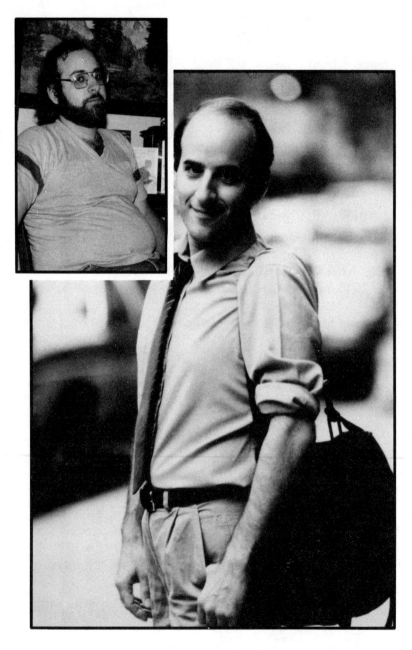

When John Passadino, a part-time comedian, learned that his weight was no joke, he decided to lighten up his act (by 67 pounds).

No More Fat Jokes

"In the next year I became a total vegetarian—excluding even dairy products. I became very fanatical about my diet. And I was trying to squeeze too much exercise into my already tight schedule. As a result, I was under a lot of stress. So I decided to relax a little, in both my diet and exercising.

"I could afford to by that point. In June 1990, when I stopped trying to lose and started trying to maintain, I weighed 138 pounds. I really looked too thin then, and not just to my mother, who insisted I was sick!

"So I put myself on a maintenance plan that I continue to follow today. I drink skim milk and eat nonfat yogurt. I eat egg whites, but still no yolks. I eat seafood twice a week—mainly tuna and salmon and sometimes scallops or shrimp.

"I relaxed my exercise program, too. Now I walk at a brisk pace four times a week for half an hour or an hour. If the weather is bad, I opt for 45 minutes on my exercise bike. And I do calisthenics three or four times a week.

"I try to stay away from sugar and alcohol. I continue to eat a low-fat diet and I focus on foods like beans and rice, rather than meats.

"The results have been great—my cholesterol fluctuates between 190 and 210. The cramping in my legs is gone and I can breathe easily now. I have a 32-inch waist, and my weight stays around 145. I'm happy to say my weight loss has actually helped, rather than hurt, my comedy. Once I lost weight, I realized I would have to rely on my talent to be funny—there was no fat to do it for me anymore. As a result, I think I'm funnier now than I ever was!"

Fighting Heredity and Winning!

Stephanie Miller never walked in front of mirrors. At 315 pounds, the 5 feet, 6 inches woman from Barstow, California, felt it reflected poorly on her. And though her weight had made her self-conscious all her life, at age 24 she suddenly discovered it was jeopardizing her health, too. Her blood pressure and cholesterol levels were sky high, and she was a borderline diabetic. That was when she decided to fight back. She started with a pinch of smart eating, and moved forward with a sampling of suitable exercise. But what really put the finishing spice into her pounds-off plan was following her own personal incentive program. The payoff? Renewed good health and permanent weight loss.

"I've been fat all my life. I ate basically anything I could get my hands on. Not so much because I was hungry, but because when I saw other people with food, I felt I had to have it. My mother was well known for her baking—cakes, sweet-potato pie, pecan pie. She also made a lot of fried chicken, corn bread and homemade ice cream.

"I had tried all the fad diets, and I would always lose weight, but I couldn't keep it off. Then on January 9, 1989, I found out I had reached 315 pounds. I was absolutely devastated. I was weighed during a visit to the doctor for a rash that was on my hand. When he saw how heavy I was, he decided to do a more thorough exam. My cholesterol was 334 and my blood pressure was 190/67—way too high. My blood sugar was high, too.

"I had always had headaches and blurry vision—I just thought it was a natural thing because of my job as a shipping assistant sitting at a computer terminal all day. But that wasn't the problem. The problem was my weight."

Large Inheritance

"Actually, my whole family is overweight. Both my mother and father have diabetes as a result, and my father had already lost several toes because of the disease. So I took the doctor's warning seriously. I felt more motivated than ever before. The doctor told me that I had to lose at least 50 pounds, and he gave me a 1,200-calorie-a-day diet.

"When I returned to work from my doctor's appointment, I talked about it with some coworkers in the office. We decided to start a 'weight pool' and see who could lose the most in six weeks. I know it's dangerous and we shouldn't have done it, but we all started out on a drastic diet, much lower than the 1,200 calories a day. I lost 22 pounds in 14 days, which won the weight pool.

"Soon after I had lost some weight, I bought myself my first pair of stone-washed jeans. It felt so good that I decided to keep going with the weight loss, but to be safe, I shifted to the sensible diet my doctor had recommended."

No Chewing the Fat

"I ate a low-fat diet of mostly chicken, fish and turkey, a lot of raw vegetables, cooked vegetables and salads. I still used some fats, such as mayonnaise, but I measured out very small portions. I also gave up fried food—all my meals were baked, broiled or roasted.

"I wanted to start exercising, too, but I was too self-conscious to go to the gym. Then I got the idea to start walking 30 minutes during my lunch break. I didn't get too far at first, but each day I tried to increase the distance. When I had lost 30 pounds, I started walking a whole hour and 15 minutes after work. After I lost 50 pounds, I joined an aerobics class. It was difficult because everybody else in there had a perfect body, it seemed to me. But I stood in the back and just walked through the motions at first. After

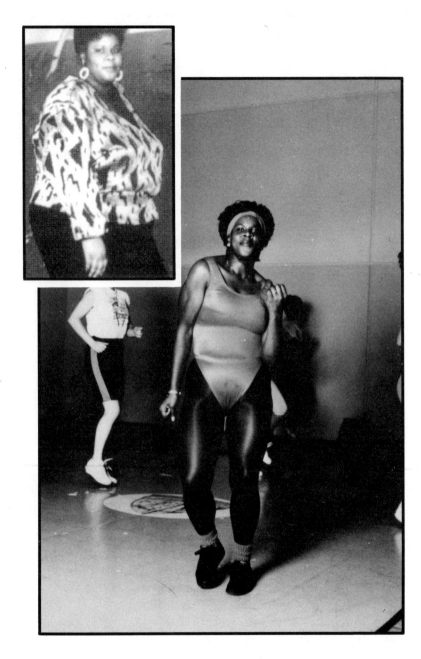

Stephanie Miller lost 153 pounds in 19 months using positive reinforcement, aerobics and a low-fat diet.

about three months, I was able to start jumping a little bit. Eventually I got to where I could do the whole routine. But believe it or not, my biggest concern about losing weight did not involve diet or exercise. My biggest concern was how my husband would react to the new me. He's in the army and was stationed in Germany while I awaited assignment of family housing. I had mixed emotions because I thought he loved me fat. (I weighed 275 pounds when we got married.)

"We were separated for eight months before the housing came through, and by the time I was ready to meet him in Germany, I had lost 90 pounds. I felt really good about myself, and I was hoping and praying that my husband would feel the same way. When I got to the airport in Germany, I waited for him with a camera in my hand, because everybody wanted me to take his picture when he saw me. But he walked right by—he didn't even recognize me!

"Finally I walked up to him, tapped him on the back and said, 'Hi.' He said, 'Hi,' then turned away and kept looking around the airport. About five seconds later, he realized his mistake, turned back and said, 'Stephanie, is that you? What happened to you?'

"I said, 'I decided you deserve a smaller wife.' And for the first time in our married life, my husband picked me up and hugged me."

Getting Back on Track

"The transition to living in Germany was very difficult for me. I got very depressed and started to overeat again. I quickly gained three pounds.

"But I sat myself down and told myself that I had worked too hard to get where I was. I couldn't give in.

"I went to a dietitian for help and got back on my 1,200-calorie diet. I joined a support group and started exercising again. I also learned to check my progress by taking my measurements rather than hopping on a scale. When I noticed that although I wasn't always losing weight, I was losing inches, I set my goals accordingly.

"When I accomplished these goals, I'd reward myself with gifts. I'd buy a novel or a blouse—anything to say, 'I deserve that. I worked hard for it.' That really helped me keep going and the weight continued to come off.

Winning at Losing

"I'm really delighted with my current weight of 164. I went from size 46 jeans to a size 11. I lost inches everywhere on my body—even my ring size dropped from 11 to 6.

"I do aerobics and ride a stationary bike five days a week now and use strength-training machines twice a week. But Saturdays and Sundays are reserved for walking.

"I eventually want to get my weight down to 130 pounds. The key to losing now seems to be patience. While I was losing eight to ten pounds a month in the beginning, now I'm losing only four to five pounds a month.

"But I stick with it and my life keeps changing for the better. Now I walk by mirrors at every opportunity. And I enjoy wearing makeup—something I'd never done before because I felt people would think I was a big clown. I don't mind sitting down on the floor any more, because now I can get back up without help.

"My health has improved, too. My blood pressure is down to 120/80 and my cholesterol is down to 198—both back in the normal range. I don't get any headaches or blurry vision, though I'm now doing the same job I was doing in the States. But best of all, now that I'm in control of both my blood pressure and weight, I look forward to starting a family.

"I keep a picture of the old me on my refrigerator. I never intend to look like that again."

Striding Himself Slim

Quitting smoking was a big step for 47-year-old *David Leek* of Davenport, Iowa. But it wasn't quite big enough. A couple of years after quitting, with his blood pressure still on the rise, his doctor gave him an ultimatum: Lose weight or take a higher dosage of blood pressure medication. David rose to the challenge again. At the suggestion of some helpful relatives, he dedicated himself to learning a whole new way of walking. By stepping up his stride, he was able to trample down his blood pressure. Coupled with a touch of smarter eating, his new pastime left him 33 pounds lighter, with a slimmer waistline and a lower cholesterol level as well.

"In 1985, at 41 years of age, I quit smoking for the last time. I had smoked filterless cigarettes since I was 15 years old, and I was seeing myself deteriorate.

"My blood pressure was high (140/110), and medication had brought it down only slightly to 130/100. And my cholesterol level was somewhat high, too: 220. I had severe headaches—at least three a week. I was wheezing, and I couldn't walk quickly without losing my breath. I believed that smoking was going to kill me.

"I quit smoking in an effort to avoid a heart attack. My dad had died from a heart condition and I felt that genetics were against me. But I also believe my dad's heart condition was a product of his bad habits of overeating and smoking—which I'd also 'inherited.'

"I assumed that quitting smoking would lower my blood pressure, relieving me of the medication I'd been on for three years. But 2½ years after quitting, my blood pressure continued to rise. At 5 feet, 7 inches and 193 pounds, my doctor told me if I didn't lose weight, he would have to raise the dosage. Although my wheezing and headaches had subsided since I'd quit smoking, I still needed to lower my blood pressure. My doctor had recommended exercise,

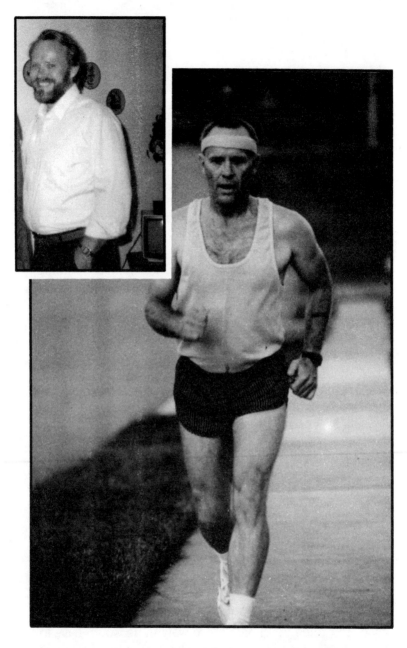

Race walking, quitting smoking and a low-fat diet helped David Leek beat a path to permanent weight loss and a healthy heart.

and two of my wife's relatives encouraged me to try race walking. Reluctantly, I joined a race walking group with them."

Best Foot Forward

"It was very difficult for me at first. It took me about six months to learn race walking technique. At first I walked five days a week, averaging about three miles a day at a 16- or 17-minute-mile pace. On Saturday mornings, our group walked for about an hour on a path that borders the Mississippi River and runs about 6.2 miles—half along the river and half along a golf course. Gradually, I built up to where I could race walk the whole course.

"Almost immediately, I began to notice changes in the way I felt. Before I started walking, I felt tired all the time. Suddenly, I had an intense energy level. After six months, my blood pressure came down enough (110/80) that my doctor took me off medication. And I lost weight, too—about 35 pounds in the first year. Then I got interested in walking competitively. But I felt I needed to lose more weight to do that."

Shaping Up His Diet

"I knew from reading about health that my diet wasn't very good. I used to eat a couple of doughnuts for breakfast, and at midmorning I'd eat anything I could get my hands on—usually a pastry. For lunch, I ate bologna sandwiches on white bread and drank soda. And every now and then I'd go on a cupcake binge. I couldn't just eat one—I'd eat half a dozen!

"So I started eating a healthy, whole-grain breakfast cereal with fruit and orange juice. Now I eat all whole-wheat breads and drink skim milk. I cut down on fatty red meats and eat leaner ones, and I eat chicken or turkey without the skin. I have a very low fat intake, and I am careful to eat in moderation.

"Coupled with walking, my new eating habits helped me shed another eight pounds. I did try race walking in several competitions. But because I'd had an operation on my right leg several years before, my form was far from impeccable and I often was disqualified. As a result, I don't race competitively anymore. But I didn't get turned off to race walking.

"On the contrary, I've been race walking for about 2½ years now, averaging five miles a day, five days a week. And I've improved. I'm probably doing about an 11-minute mile now.

"I put back a little weight when I stopped racing competitively, but my improved eating habits have helped me maintain myself at 160 pounds for over a year now.

"Knowing that I was feeling better physically enhanced the way I felt psychologically, too. And watching myself slide into a pair of blue jeans that two years previously I couldn't even zip up—that was a big boost! What probably helped me most, though, were the flattering comments from those in my race walking group who encouraged me along the way."

Finding Time to Live

"People say, 'I just don't have time in my schedule to walk.' Well, I said I didn't have time. But the reality of it is, when something does go wrong, when you see your health deteriorating, then you make the time. I'm just sorry I waited until something was wrong.

"I'm able to do so much more now. My energy and endurance levels are higher. I enjoy doing yard work and other work around the house. I get up in the morning feeling well rested because I'm sleeping better. And I can't wait to get home from work and go for my walk.

"My blood pressure is now 115/70 and my cholesterol has dropped to 170. I continue to walk no matter what the weather—sun, rain or snow. And I now ride a mountain bike to work (12 miles, round-trip) three times a week, weather permitting. I found in order to change my life, I had to actively live it. Now I do have time for my health."

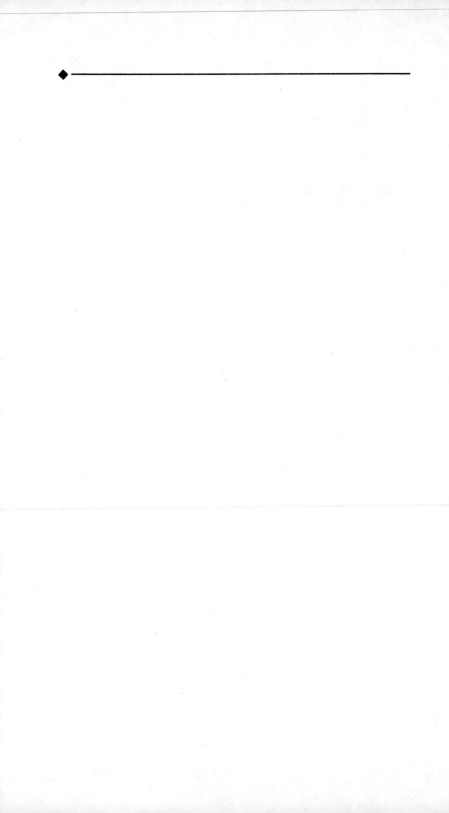

CHAPTER

SAVOR THE FLAVOR WITHOUT THE FAT: THE YUMMIEST, EASIEST LIGHT RECIPES OF THE YEAR

What's a dieter's worst enemy? Calories? Dietary fat? Lack of willpower? No! Certainly, all those things conspire to put on pounds and keep them there. But a dieter's worst enemy is a "diet" that doesn't taste good, one that doesn't really satisfy both physical hunger and a psychological need for visually appealing food. That's why delicious, healthful food has become a priority for a successful weight-loss plan.

Here are some of today's most delicious, healthy recipes—low in cholesterol and sodium, and packed with fiber and good nutrition. Best of all, each contains 25 percent or less of calories from fat. Good news whether you're concerned about heart disease, cancer or your weight! So eat up. This healthy fare is definitely worth savoring.

Power-Packed Breakfasts in a Flash

Broccoli Frittata

    ½ small onion, chopped
    1 tablespoon olive oil
    1 cup chopped frozen broccoli (no need to thaw)
    1 tablespoon minced fresh herbs, such as basil or
       dill
    1 cup egg substitute or 8 egg whites
    ½ cup low-fat cottage cheese

In a large frying pan over medium heat, sauté the onions in the oil for 5 minutes, or until soft. Add the broccoli and herbs; sauté for a few minutes.

In a small bowl, whisk together the eggs and cottage cheese. Pour over the broccoli. Stir a few times to blend. Cook for 3 to 5 minutes.

Transfer to the oven and bake at 350° for about 15 minutes, or until the eggs are set.

Serves 4

Per serving: 92 calories, 2.5 grams fat (24 percent of calories), 2 grams dietary fiber, 12.6 grams protein, 2 milligrams cholesterol, 238 milligrams sodium. Also a good source of vitamins A and C.

Golden Carrot Bars

         2 cups rolled oats
         1 cup ready-to-eat cereal flakes
         1 cup whole-wheat pastry flour
         1 tablespoon baking powder
         1 cup shredded carrots
        ½ cup raisins
         1 teaspoon ground cinnamon
         1 cup water
        ½ cup instant nonfat dry milk
        ½ cup maple syrup
         2 egg whites
         2 tablespoons canola or lightly flavored olive oil

In a large bowl, combine the oats, cereal flakes, flour and baking powder. Stir in the carrots, raisins and cinnamon.

In a medium bowl, whisk together the water and dry milk until smooth. Whisk in the maple syrup, egg whites and oil. Pour over the dry ingredients. Mix until just combined; do not overmix. Let stand 10 minutes.

Coat a 9″ × 13″ baking dish with no-stick spray. Pour in the batter and level the top with a spatula. Bake at 350° for 25 to 35 minutes, or until firm to the touch. Turn off the heat and leave the pan in the oven, with the door ajar, for 2 hours. Cut into bars.

Makes 10 bars
Per bar: 226 calories, 4.1 grams fat (16 percent of calories), 3.8 grams dietary fiber, 7 grams protein, 1 milligram cholesterol, 186 milligrams sodium. Also a good source of vitamin A.

Pineapple Spoon Bread

1¼   cups yellow cornmeal
¾   cup unbleached flour
1   tablespoon baking powder
1   cup buttermilk
2   egg whites
2   tablespoons maple syrup
2   tablespoons canola or lightly flavored olive oil
10   pineapple rings or 1½ cups chopped pineapple

In a large bowl, mix the dry ingredients.

In a medium bowl, whisk together the buttermilk, egg whites, maple syrup and 1 tablespoon of the oil. Pour over the dry ingredients and mix until just combined; do not overmix.

Coat a 10½-inch cast-iron skillet with no-stick spray. Spoon in the batter. Level with a spatula and arrange the pineapple rings or chopped pineapple on top. Brush with the remaining 1 tablespoon oil.

Bake at 400° for 18 minutes, or until the bread has begun to pull away from the sides of the pan and a tooth-pick inserted in the center comes out clean.

Slice into wedges and serve topped with additional pineapple (optional).

Serves 6
Per serving: 245 calories, 6 grams fat (22 percent of calories), 3.6 grams dietary fiber, 6.5 grams protein, 1.5 milligrams cholesterol, 232 milligrams sodium.

Lean Bean Lunch Salads

Lentil and Pea Salad
with Scallion Vinaigrette

     4½ tablespoons extra-virgin olive oil
     ¼   cup red-wine vinegar
     1   tablespoon Dijon mustard
     1   clove garlic, minced
     ¼   teaspoon ground black pepper
     2   cups dried brown or French lentils
     1   bay leaf
     1   thick slice onion
     1   leafy celery top
     1   clove garlic, lightly crushed
     1   cup diced celery
     1   cup cooked and cooled peas
     ⅔   cup thinly sliced scallions
     ½   cup minced fresh flat-leaf parsley
     ¼   cup diced sweet red peppers

In a large bowl, whisk together the oil, vinegar, mustard, minced garlic and black pepper. Set aside.

Sort and rinse the lentils. Place them in a 3-quart saucepan with the bay leaf, onion slice, celery top and crushed garlic. Add about 8 cups of cold water. Bring to a boil. Cook uncovered over medium heat, stirring frequently, for about 15 minutes, or until the lentils are tender.

Take 1 tablespoon of cooking water and whisk into the dressing in the bowl. Drain lentils and discard bay leaf, onion, celery and garlic.

Transfer the warm lentils to the bowl and lightly fold to coat them with the dressing. Fold in the diced celery, peas, scallions, parsley and red peppers. Serve chilled or at room temperature.

Serves 6

Per serving: 378 calories, 11 grams fat (25 percent of calories), 11 grams dietary fiber, 23.2 grams protein, no cholesterol, 84 milligrams sodium. Also a good source of thiamine, vitamin C and iron.

Three-Bean Salad

1½   cups dried red beans, soaked overnight
1   bay leaf
1   leafy celery top
1   thick slice onion
1   clove garlic, lightly crushed
¼   cup sherry vinegar or fruit vinegar
2   tablespoons white vinegar
3   tablespoons extra-virgin olive oil
1   clove garlic, minced
¼   teaspoon ground black pepper
12   ounces fresh wax beans
12   ounces fresh green beans
⅔   cup diced cucumbers
½   cup thinly sliced scallions
¼   cup minced fresh flat-leaf parsley

Drain the soaked red beans and transfer them to a 3-quart saucepan. Add the bay leaf, celery top, onion slice and crushed garlic. Add about 8 cups of cold water. Bring to a boil. Simmer uncovered over medium heat, stirring occasionally, for 1 to 1½ hours, or until the beans are tender.

While the beans are cooking, combine the vinegars, oil, minced garlic and pepper in a large bowl. Set aside.

When the beans are tender, spoon out 2 tablespoons of the cooking water and whisk it into the dressing mixture in the bowl. Drain the beans well and discard the bay leaf, celery, onion and garlic. Add the warm beans to the dressing and stir lightly. Set aside to cool.

Trim the wax beans and green beans. Cut into ¾-inch pieces. Blanch in a large pot of boiling water for 3 to 5 minutes, or until tender. Drain the beans and rinse them in cold water. Set aside.

Just before serving, add the wax beans, green beans, cucumbers, scallions and parsley to the red beans. Stir lightly to blend. Serve at room temperature.

Serves 6
Per serving: 270 calories, 7.6 grams fat (24 percent of calories), 7.1 grams dietary fiber, 14 grams protein, no cholesterol, 12 milligrams sodium. Also a good source of thiamine, vitamin C and iron.

Black-Eyed Peas and Carrots with Tarragon Dressing

1⅓	cups dried black-eyed peas, soaked overnight
1	bay leaf
1	thick slice onion
1	sprig fresh tarragon
1	clove garlic, lightly crushed
¼	cup white-wine vinegar
2 ½	tablespoons extra-virgin olive oil
2	tablespoons lemon juice
2	tablespoons minced fresh tarragon
1	tablespoon snipped chives
¼	teaspoon ground black pepper
2	cups diced carrots
½	cup diced green peppers
½	cup diced red onions

Drain the black-eyed peas and transfer them to a
3-quart saucepan. Add the bay leaf, onion slice, tarragon
sprig and garlic. Add about 8 cups of cold water. Bring to
a boil. Simmer uncovered over medium heat, stirring
occasionally, for about 1 hour or until the peas are tender.

In a large bowl, whisk together the vinegar, oil,
lemon juice, minced tarragon, chives and black pepper.
Set aside.

While the peas are cooking, blanch the carrots in
boiling water for 3 minutes, or until crisp. Drain and add
to the bowl with the dressing. Stir well and set aside.

When the peas are tender, spoon out 3 tablespoons
of the cooking water and add it to the carrot mixture.
Drain the peas and discard the bay leaf, onion, tarragon
and garlic.

Combine peas and carrots and stir lightly to blend.
Add the green peppers and red onions. Toss well. Serve
chilled or at room temperature.

Serves 6
*Per serving: 257 calories, 7.1 grams fat (24 percent of
calories), 12.5 grams dietary fiber, 14.2 grams protein, no
cholesterol, 31 milligrams sodium. Also a good source of
thiamine, vitamins A and C and potassium.*

Skinny Simmered Suppers

*Chicken Meatballs
with Tomato-Basil Sauce*

Chicken Meatballs
1 pound extra-lean ground chicken
¼ cup finely diced onions

   ¼ cup dry bread crumbs
   1 egg white
   2 teaspoons low-sodium soy sauce
   ¼ teaspoon dried oregano
   ¼ teaspoon dried basil
   1 clove garlic, minced

Tomato-Basil Sauce
   6 large ripe tomatoes
   ½ cup red-wine vinegar
1½ cups defatted chicken stock
   2 yellow peppers, julienned
   2 green peppers, julienned
   1 red onion, julienned
   2 ounces fresh basil, chopped
   3 cloves garlic, finely chopped
   ½ teaspoon dried oregano

   8 ounces pasta

To make the meatballs: In a large bowl, mix together the chicken, onions, bread crumbs, egg white, soy sauce, oregano, basil and garlic. Form mixture into 12 meatballs. Place on a no-stick baking sheet. Bake at 350° for 25 minutes.

To make the tomato-basil sauce: On a grill or under a broiler, char the tomatoes until they are blackened on all sides. Remove the peels and coarsely chop the flesh. (You should end up with about 4 cups of flesh and juice.) Transfer to a Dutch oven. Add the vinegar, stock, yellow peppers, green peppers, onion, basil, garlic and oregano. Simmer over medium heat for 30 minutes.

While the sauce is cooking, cook the pasta in a large pot of boiling water until just tender (the exact time will depend upon the type of pasta you've used). Drain and place in a large serving bowl. Top with the sauce and meatballs.

Serves 4

Per serving: 539 calories, 14.8 grams fat (25 percent of calories), 4.6 grams dietary fiber, 33 grams protein, 80 milligrams cholesterol, 267 milligrams sodium. Also a very good source of vitamin C and thiamine and a good source of vitamin A, riboflavin, niacin, potassium and iron.

Warm Chicken Salad with Roasted Garlic Vinaigrette

Marinated Cucumbers and Onions

  1 cup rice-wine vinegar
  1 teaspoon honey
 ⅛ teaspoon red-pepper flakes
  1 cucumber, thinly sliced on the diagonal
  1 red onion, thinly sliced

Roasted Garlic Vinaigrette

  8 cloves garlic, unpeeled
  2 large ripe tomatoes, peeled, seeded and chopped
 ½ cup red-wine vinegar
  1 tablespoon minced fresh basil
  1 teaspoon minced fresh oregano
  1 teaspoon dried basil
 ½ teaspoon dried oregano

Marinated Chicken Breasts

  1 tablespoon lemon juice
  1 clove garlic, minced
  1 teaspoon olive oil
 ¼ teaspoon dried oregano
  4 boneless skinless chicken breast halves
  8 fresh shiitake mushrooms

Assembly

4 cups torn lettuce or other greens

To make the marinated cucumbers and onions: In a large bowl, combine the vinegar, honey and pepper flakes. Add the cucumber and onion; toss to coat. Allow to marinate for 2 hours.

To make the roasted garlic vinaigrette: Place the garlic in a custard cup. Cover with foil and bake at 450° for 20 minutes, or until tender and lightly browned. Let cool slightly, then remove the cloves from their peels. Place the garlic in a blender. Add the tomatoes, vinegar, fresh basil, fresh oregano, dried basil and dried oregano. Process until smooth. Set aside.

To make the marinated chicken breasts: In a small cup, combine the lemon juice, minced garlic, olive oil and oregano. Rub over all sides of the chicken. Place the breasts on a baking sheet. Remove and discard the stems from the mushrooms. Place the mushrooms on the sheet. Bake at 450° for 8 to 10 minutes. Remove from the oven and slice the chicken on the bias.

To assemble the salad: Place the lettuce or greens in a large bowl. Process the vinaigrette for a few seconds to recombine the ingredients. Pour over the greens and toss well. Divide among 4 dinner plates.

Drain the cucumber and onion; arrange next to the greens. Place chicken and mushrooms over greens.

Serves 4
Per serving: 218 calories, 3.2 grams fat (13 percent of calories), 3 grams dietary fiber, 29.5 grams protein, 66 milligrams cholesterol, 90 milligrams sodium. Also a very good source of niacin, vitamin B$_6$, vitamin C and a good source of vitamin A.

Chicken with Polenta Dumplings

Day 1
1 large fennel bulb
1 chicken (about 3 pounds)
8 cups water
1 onion, halved
1 clove garlic, crushed
1 leafy celery top
6 fennel seeds
1 bay leaf

Day 2
1 can (14 ounces) Italian tomatoes, drained, seeded and coarsely chopped
¼ teaspoon ground black pepper
2 strips orange rind, julienned
⅔ cup unbleached flour
½ cup finely ground yellow cornmeal
2 teaspoons grated Parmesan cheese (optional)
1 teaspoon baking powder
  Pinch of ground red pepper
⅓ cup skim milk
1 egg white

On Day 1: Remove some of the feathery tops from the fennel; cut into 1-inch lengths, wrap well and refrigerate to use as garnish. Chop enough of the remaining fennel greens and tough outer ribs to equal ½ cup; place in a Dutch oven. Trim the remaining fennel bulb and cut into 6 lengthwise wedges; wrap well and refrigerate.

Remove and discard any visible fat from the chicken, especially from the cavity. Place the chicken in the Dutch oven. Add the water, onion, garlic, celery, fennel seeds and bay leaf. Bring to a boil, then reduce the heat to low. Simmer, uncovered, for 2 hours, or until the chicken is tender.

Transfer the chicken to a plate and let stand until cool enough to handle. Remove and discard the skin and bones. Leave the meat in large pieces. Cover and refrigerate overnight.

Strain the stock into a large bowl; discard the vegetables and bay leaf. Cover and refrigerate overnight.

On Day 2: Using a spoon or metal spatula, lift off and discard the fat that has congealed on the top of the stock.

Pour the stock into a Dutch oven. Add the fennel wedges, cover and cook over medium-low heat for 20 minutes, or until easily pierced with the tip of a knife. Add the tomatoes, black pepper, orange rind and cooked chicken. Heat through.

While the fennel is cooking, combine the flour, cornmeal, Parmesan, baking powder and red pepper in a medium bowl. In a cup whisk together the milk and egg white. Pour over the dry ingredients and stir gently with a fork until evenly moistened.

Using the tip of a tablespoon, drop 12 dumplings onto the surface of the simmering stock. Cover and simmer for 20 minutes; do not uncover during this time.

With a slotted spoon, transfer the dumplings to a plate. Divide the chicken and vegetables among six shallow soup bowls. Pour some stock into each. Top each portion with 2 dumplings. Garnish with the reserved fennel tops.

Serves 6
Per serving: 251 calories, 2 grams fat (7 percent of calories), 2 grams dietary fiber, 35 grams protein, 94 milligrams cholesterol, 220 milligrams sodium. Also a very good source of vitamin C and niacin.

Braised Beef with Vegetables

    1 pound lean eye of round steak
    1 tablespoon unbleached flour
    1 tablespoon mild paprika
    1 tablespoon herbal salt substitute
    1 teaspoon ground black pepper
    ½ cup plus 2 tablespoons water
    1 tablespoon balsamic vinegar
    1 large onion, diced
    1 cup thinly sliced carrots
    1 teaspoon caraway seeds
    2 cups halved mushrooms
    1 cup defatted beef stock
    1 tablespoon tomato paste
    8 ounces broad noodles

Place the steak in the freezer until partially frozen, about 20 minutes. Trim off all visible fat. Cut the meat into 2-inch pieces.

In a paper bag, combine the flour, paprika, salt substitute and black pepper. Shake well. Add the meat and shake again to coat the meat thoroughly. Set aside.

In a Dutch oven over medium-high heat, bring 2 tablespoons of the water and the vinegar to a boil. Add the onion, stir briskly and cook for 2 minutes. Stir in the carrots and caraway seeds; cook for 2 minutes. Stir in the mushrooms; cook for 1 minute. Transfer the vegetables to a plate.

In the same pan, bring the remaining ½ cup water to a boil. Add the meat, reduce the heat to medium and cook for about 5 minutes, stirring occasionally. Add the cooked vegetables, stock and tomato paste. Bring the mixture to a boil.

Transfer to the oven. Partially cover the pan with a lid. Bake at 350° for 1½ hours, stirring occasionally, until the meat is tender.

Cook the noodles in a large pot of boiling water until tender, about 10 minutes. Drain and place on a serving platter. Top with the meat mixture.

Serves 4
Per serving: 426 calories, 7.2 grams fat (15 percent of calories), 2.6 grams dietary fiber, 32.5 grams protein, 58 milligrams cholesterol, 77 milligrams sodium. Also a very good source of B vitamins.

Savory Herb-and-Garlic Pork Chops

    2 pork loin chops (1½ pounds)
    1 tablespoon minced garlic (optional)
    1 teaspoon ground cumin
    1 teaspoon herbal salt substitute (optional)
    ½ teaspoon ground coriander
    ¼ teaspoon ground red pepper
    ¼ teaspoon ground black pepper
    2 baking potatoes
    1 cup unsweetened applesauce
    1 cup braised red cabbage

Place the chops in the freezer until partially frozen, about 20 minutes. Trim off all visible fat.

In a cup, combine the garlic, cumin, salt substitute, coriander, red pepper and black pepper. Spread the mixture thickly on both sides of the chops. Place on a plate, cover with plastic wrap and refrigerate from 2 to 8 hours.

About 1 hour before serving, place potatoes in the oven at 350°.

Place the chops on a broiler rack and broil about 4 inches from the heat for 8 to 12 minutes per side, or until the chops are browned and crusty. Be careful not to overcook the chops so they don't dry out. When ready, serve with baked potatoes, applesauce and cabbage.

Serves 2

Per serving: 375 calories, 9.5 grams fat (23 percent of calories), 2.7 grams dietary fiber, 30 grams protein, 65 milligrams cholesterol, 74 milligrams sodium. Also a very good source of B vitamins, vitamin C and iron.

Streamlined Seafood

Fish and Corn Chowder

 2　teaspoons olive oil
 1　cup chopped onions
 ⅔　cup chopped sweet red peppers
 ½　cup chopped celery
 1　jalapeño pepper, chopped
 2　cups white corn (see Note)
 1　cup chopped tomatoes
 ½　teaspoon fresh thyme
 ¼　teaspoon ground black pepper
 2　cups chicken or fish stock
 8　ounces new potatoes, cubed
12　ounces cod or flounder fillets, cut into 1-inch pieces
1¼　cups evaporated skim milk
 1　tablespoon snipped chives

In a 3- or 4-quart pot over medium heat, warm the oil. Add the chopped onions and cook for 5 minutes, or until soft. Add the sweet red peppers, chopped celery and jalapeño pepper; cook for about 5 minutes.

Add the corn, tomatoes, thyme and black pepper. Cook for 10 minutes, stirring often to prevent sticking. Add the stock and potatoes. Bring to a boil, then reduce the heat a bit and simmer for 15 to 20 minutes, or until the potatoes are tender.

Using a slotted spoon, remove about half of the vegetables and transfer to a blender. Add about ½ cup of the liquid. Process until puréed. Pour back into the pot.

Over low heat, stir in the fish and 1 cup of the milk. Cook for about 5 minutes, or until the fish becomes just opaque. If the soup is too thick, thin with a bit of the remaining milk. Sprinkle with the chives.

Serves 4
Per serving: 308 calories, 4.9 grams fat (14 percent of calories), 7.7 grams dietary fiber, 24.9 grams protein, 38 milligrams cholesterol, 283 milligrams sodium. Also a good source of vitamin A, vitamin C, potassium and fiber.

NOTE: This chowder is best made with fresh corn. You'll need about 3 cobs. Slice off the kernels with a sharp knife, then use the back of a knife to scrape out all the remaining corn and its juice.

King Crab and Mango Salad on Corn Bread

    2 king crab legs, frozen (see Note)
   ½ cup chopped sweet red peppers
   ¼ cup chopped onions
   ¼ cup chopped fresh basil
    1 ripe mango, cubed
    2 tablespoons lime juice
    1 tablespoon balsamic vinegar
    1 tablespoon olive oil
   ½ teaspoon low-sodium soy sauce
   ½ teaspoon sesame seeds
    8 small slices or 4 squares corn bread (see Note)
   ½ head Bibb lettuce, torn into bite-sized pieces

Thaw the crab legs. Using a nutcracker or small mallet, crack the crab legs and carefully remove the meat. Break the meat into large pieces and place in a large bowl. Add the sweet red peppers, onions, basil and mango. Toss gently to combine.

In a small bowl, whisk together the lime juice, vinegar, oil and soy sauce. Pour over the crab mixture and toss to coat. Sprinkle with the sesame seeds.

Divide the corn bread among dinner plates. Top with the lettuce and the salad. Eat as open-faced sandwiches.

Serves 4

Per serving: 527 calories, 15 grams fat (25 percent of calories), 10.8 grams dietary fiber, 23.8 grams protein, 57 milligrams cholesterol, 591 milligrams sodium. Also a good source of thiamine, vitamin B_{12}, vitamin C.

NOTE: You may substitute other seafood for the crab. Cooked snow crab, scallops, lobster or chunks of white fish are all good. You may even choose surimi, the imitation form of crab, lobster and shrimp that's becoming popular. As for the corn bread, use your favorite recipe.

Tuna Blue-Plate Special

12-ounce tuna fillet, 1 inch thick
¼ cup sherry vinegar or cider vinegar
2 tablespoons lemon juice
1 tablespoon snipped chives or minced fresh basil
2 teaspoons low-sodium soy sauce
1 clove garlic, minced
¼ teaspoon ground red pepper
1 tablespoon olive oil
3 carrots, cut into ½″ × 2″ pieces

3   parsnips, cut into ½″ × 2″ pieces
2   onions, quartered
1   teaspoon fresh rosemary
1   teaspoon fresh thyme
8   small new potatoes
1   whole garlic bulb
8   slices whole-grain bread
    Nonfat mayonnaise, tomatoes, lettuce (optional)

Wash the tuna and pat it dry.

In a shallow dish, whisk together the vinegar, lemon juice, chives or basil, soy sauce, minced garlic and pepper. Add the tuna and turn to coat both sides. Refrigerate and allow to marinate for about 1 hour.

Coat the bottom of a 9″ × 13″ baking dish with 1 teaspoon of the oil. Add the carrots, parsnips, onions, rosemary and thyme. Pare a strip of peel from each potato; add the potatoes to the dish. Break the garlic bulb into cloves, peel and add. Drizzle with 1 teaspoon of the remaining oil and toss to coat all the vegetables.

Roast at 400°, stirring occasionally, for about 1 hour, or until the vegetables are tender but not mushy.

About 15 minutes before the vegetables are ready, heat a well-seasoned cast-iron skillet on medium-high until hot. Add the remaining 1 teaspoon oil. Remove the tuna from the marinade, place in the pan and sear for 2 minutes per side, or until golden brown.

Coat a small baking sheet with no-stick spray. Transfer the tuna to the sheet. Place in the oven and bake with the vegetables for 7 minutes, or until medium rare. (If you prefer the tuna rare, like a steak, bake it for 6 minutes.)

Slice the tuna thinly on a bias, as you would London broil. Use the bread and your choice of condiments (such as nonfat mayonnaise, tomatoes and lettuce) to make sandwiches. Eat with the vegetables.

Serves 4

Per serving: 547 calories, 6.8 grams fat (11 percent of calories), 9 grams dietary fiber, 31.3 grams protein, 38 milligrams cholesterol, 391 milligrams sodium. Also a good source of vitamin A, thiamine, niacin, folate, vitamin B_6, vitamin C, potassium.

Grilled Bass with Ginger

    4   skinless bass fillets (6 ounces each)
    1   lemon, quartered lengthwise
    2   cloves garlic, minced
    ½   teaspoon ground black pepper
    1   medium zucchini
    1   medium yellow squash
    1   small carrot, julienned
    1   parsnip, julienned
    2   tablespoons minced fresh ginger

Season the bass by squeezing lemon juice over both sides of each fillet. Sprinkle with the garlic and pepper. Set aside for 15 to 20 minutes.

Cut the zucchini and squash into 2-inch chunks. Core each piece to remove the seeds. Cut the remainder into julienne pieces. Place in a large bowl. Add the carrot, parsnip and ginger. Toss lightly to combine. Set aside.

Cut 4 large pieces of foil (16 inches × 16 inches). Fold each in half to make a double thickness. Divide the vegetables into 4 portions and place 1 portion on half of each piece of foil. Top with the fish.

Fold the foil over the fish and crimp the edges to tightly seal the packets.

Grill over medium-high heat for 15 to 20 minutes. If desired, serve right in the foil.

Serves 4

Per serving: 244 calories, 8.7 grams fat, 1.7 grams die-tary fiber, 34 grams protein, 116 milligrams cholesterol, 130 milligrams sodium. Also a good source of thiamine, vitamin C, calcium, iron.

Steamed Ginger Salmon

1   pound salmon fillet
3   tablespoons mirin (Japanese cooking wine)
2   tablespoons chopped fresh ginger
2   tablespoons low-sodium soy sauce
2   tablespoons minced scallions
4   cloves garlic, minced
1   teaspoon honey
¼   teaspoon hot-pepper sauce
3   cups hot cooked rice
1   piece (1 inch) fresh ginger, julienned
    Coriander sprigs

Rinse the salmon and pat it dry. Cut into 4 to 6 pieces. Remove any bones (use tweezers).

In a shallow dish, whisk together the mirin, chopped ginger, soy sauce, scallions, garlic, honey and hot-pepper sauce. Add the salmon and turn to coat both sides. Refrigerate and allow to marinate for 1 hour.

Remove the fish from the marinade and place it in a large steamer basket; reserve the marinade. Steam the fish for about 7 minutes, or until it flakes if stabbed with a fork and the interior is dark red.

Place the rice on a serving platter. Add the fish and sprinkle with the julienned ginger and coriander sprigs; keep warm.

Strain the marinade into a 1-quart saucepan. Bring to a full boil and remove from heat. Serve with the fish as a dipping sauce.

Serves 4

Per serving: 343 calories, 8.6 grams fat (23 percent of calories), 2.6 grams dietary fiber, 27.5 grams protein, 63 milligrams cholesterol, 360 milligrams sodium. Also a good source of niacin, vitamin B_6, vitamin B_{12}, potassium.

NOTE: An alternate way to steam the fish is in a wok. Bring an inch of water to a boil in the wok. Add a bamboo basket or cake rack. Place the fish and its marinade in a glass pie plate and place on the rack. Cover with a lid and steam as directed above.

Broiled Scallops and Grapefruit

  1   pound large sea scallops
  2   pink grapefruits
  2   tablespoons snipped chives
16   ounces kale
  2   teaspoons hazelnut oil or olive oil
  2   cloves garlic

Rinse the scallops and pat dry. Slice each scallop in half horizontally. Place in a large glass bowl.

Working over the bowl (to catch all the juices), peel and section the grapefruit. Add the sections to the scallops. Squeeze the leftover membranes to extract as much juice as possible. Add the chives and toss gently to combine. Refrigerate and allow scallops to marinate for 1 hour.

Meanwhile, wash and trim the kale and break into small pieces. Drain in a colander, but don't shake off the excess water; it will help to steam-cook the kale later. Set aside.

Place the scallops and grapefruit in a shallow pan. Broil, close to the heat, for 3 minutes. Flip the pieces and broil for 2 minutes.

Heat the oil in a large no-stick frying pan over medium heat. Add the garlic and cook until golden, about 2 minutes. Discard the garlic. Add the kale to the pan and cook, stirring, until its edges start to crisp, about 4 to 6 minutes.

Divide the kale among dinner plates and top with the scallops and grapefruit.

Serves 4

Per serving: 216 calories, 4 grams fat (16 percent of calories), 1.6 grams dietary fiber, 23.6 grams protein, 37 milligrams cholesterol, 233 milligrams sodium. Also a good source of vitamin A, vitamin B_{12}, vitamin C, potassium.

Taming the Taste of Garlic

Is garlic just a little too fierce for your taste? Do you tend to avoid this pungent herb, despite scientific evidence that it may be good for you? What you need are a few tips for turning this culinary tiger into a purring kitten. Cooking garlic softens its flavor and brings out a sweetness the raw herb can't match. Unlike a quick sauté, which risks burning the garlic and uncovering an unpleasant bitterness, the methods discussed here treat it tenderly.

Parboiling. Bring some water to a boil in a small saucepan. Add unpeeled garlic cloves. Reduce the heat and simmer the garlic about 10 minutes, or until soft. Drain and slip off the skins. Mash the garlic and use in dips, spreads and salad dressings. Or mix with a little nonfat mayo or yogurt to use on grilled meat or fish.

Roasting. Take your pick of methods: Cut the very top off an entire head of garlic to expose the cloves, then loosely wrap the bulb in foil (toss in some fresh herbs if you like) and bake at 350° for about 1 hour. Or break the bulb into individual cloves and place the pieces in a custard cup with enough stock to cover. Seal the cup with foil and bake at 350° for 30 minutes, or until the cloves are tender.

Either method yields garlic with a pleasant nutty flavor. Peel the cloves and mix them with cooked vegetables. Or add the peeled cloves to pesto sauce (you can cut back on the amount of pine nuts or walnuts in the recipe). Another way to serve roasted garlic is to simply squeeze the softened clove from its peel and spread onto thick slices of crusty bread as a creamy nonfat substitute for butter.

Slow simmering. Long, slow cooking in soups and sauces also brings out garlic's best behavior. Peel the cloves and chop them coarsely. Add to tomato sauce and all types of soup. Let the mixture bubble away over gentle heat until the garlic is very soft. The fragrant steam rising from the pot has an irresistible aroma

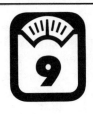

THE CONSUMER'S DETECTIVE AGENCY: A REVEALING LOOK AT THE DIET INDUSTRY

Today's weight-loss industry is big business. Diet pills, diet shakes, diet centers and many other "weight loss aids" are cropping up everywhere we look. In the face of aggressive marketing and sometimes deceptive advertising, an unsuspecting consumer can all too easily fall for "quick weight loss" scams. Diet fraud, unfortunately, is also big business.

Just how many of the heavily promoted products really work? And how safe are they? If you invest in one kind of diet program to the exclusion of all others, will it make you thin or just make your wallet thinner? Will some of those much-vaunted diet programs end up damaging your health?

This chapter is designed to help you become a judicious consumer in the weight-loss marketplace. Looking at some of the most popular services and diet aids, we'll help you detect the good and reject the good-for-nothing.

Be a Dietitian Detective: How to Pick a Pro

At least one nutritionist we know eats nothing but cat food. We're referring to Charlie, Dr. Victor Herbert's cat. Dr. Herbert, a national authority on vitamins and minerals, obtained nutrition diplomas for his pet cat and pet dog, Sassafras, by sending $50 apiece to an unaccredited school for nutritionists and a nutritional association.

It's a funny story, but the damage that has been inflicted by unqualified nutritionists isn't so funny.

The harm can be anything from death—mostly caused because someone had a deadly disease and delayed seeing a legitimate professional—to money lost from "cures" that are harmless but expensive.

But as long as you know how to weed through the

quacks, a nutritionist can help you make great changes in your diet. First, get a list of registered dietitians (R.D.) in your area by sending a self-addressed, stamped envelope to the National Center for Nutrition and Dietetics, 216 W. Jackson Blvd., Suite 800, Chicago, IL 60606–6995. Tell them you would like a copy of their Consulting Nutritionist List for your state.

"There may be good nutritionists who are not R.D.'s, but it's safer to find someone with that credential, because it means they have at least four years of college study in nutrition and a dietetic internship," says Pat Harper, a registered dietitian in the Pittsburgh area. "The term *nutritionist* has no legal definition, so almost anyone can call himself a nutritionist, even if he has no experience in the area."

Still, some R.D.'s are better than others. To find the best you can get, call a few and ask them what they can do for you. Compare your answers to our hallmarks of a pro and warning signs of a con.

What a Good Nutritionist Can Do for You

Clear up misconceptions. "Even people who know a lot about nutrition still may have gaps in their knowledge," says Mona Sutnick, a registered dietitian and spokesperson for the American Dietetic Association (ADA) who practices in Philadelphia. "They may have misconceptions about what is and isn't fattening. Or maybe they can count calories but don't know much about fiber or vitamins. A dietitian can help you develop a meal plan that takes care of all your nutritional needs."

Harper, who is also a spokesperson for the ADA, agrees. "Some people think they know enough information, but without the education and experience they may not be qualified to give accurate advice. An R.D. devotes her life to looking at details of diet and can help sort through confusing, conflicting information. And I see so many misconceptions. One common mistake people make is restricting a diet too much. Some people learn they can eat a lot more than they thought they could."

Translate doctors' advice. "Anyone who has been given a specific diet prescription by a physician should see a registered dietitian for further explanation and personalized meal plans to help you put it into practice," says Harper.

If you have diabetes, for instance, your diet will not be the same as every other diabetic's. Your doctor will give you a specific prescription based on your size, age, sex and health status. He or she will tell you how many calories, carbohydrates, fat, protein and other nutrients you can eat. You need a dietitian to help translate it into real life: what to buy at the supermarket, what to make for meals, how to cook it and how much to eat.

A dietitian can design your diet for conditions such as allergies, cancer, diabetes, hypertension, hypoglycemia, heart disease, malnutrition, obesity, pregnancy and lactation. If you can, find a dietitian who specializes in any condition you may have.

Custom-tailor your diet. "A dietitian will help you design a personalized diet, taking into consideration what foods you like and your lifestyle," says Harper. "You can't change your whole life and your food preferences so that you can follow a standard diet sheet. We help you fit a diet into your life, not fit your life into some diet."

As useful as books about nutrition may be, they just can't give everyone the personalized advice a one-on-one adviser can—that's difficult with more than 70,000 readers. "General guidelines in eating out can be helpful, but I take it one step further," says Harper. "I have my clients bring in menus from their favorite restaurants, and we discuss which dishes are best."

Do a follow-up. After you work out an eating plan with your dietitian, you will go out in the real world and find out whether you can live with the plan. Chances are, there will be parts of your diet you can't live with. "That's why you need a follow-up," says Sutnick. "I try to keep in account what my client can and can't do, and we modify the plan to make it more 'doable.' In my practice, we usually have weekly consultations until the person knows what he's doing."

Make house calls, if necessary. Some dietitians make home visits to people who are homebound because of a disease or disability. They assess the client's current food supplies, cooking facilities and cooking capabilities and tailor advice to their lifestyle, food preferences, nutritional needs and budget. This kind of service is more expensive and isn't available in all parts of the country.

Tip-Offs to a Bogus Nutritionist

A qualified nutritionist would not:

• Hand out preprinted diet sheets without giving individualized advice.
• Promise that weight loss will be quick, easy and effortless.
• Advise you not to eat certain food groups or tell you to eat large amounts of a particular type of food.
• Prescribe megadoses of supplements.
• Evaluate nutritional status by fingernail, hair or saliva analysis.
• Sell products and supplements they recommend.
• Recommend you buy only one particular brand of food, without giving a choice.
• Recommend a diet with less than 1,000 calories a day, unless in specific cases and under a doctor's supervision.
• Promise to cure chronic diseases.

War of the Diets: The Weight-Loss Centers Are Battling for Customers
By Joanne Silberner

It was a battle that Representative Ron Wyden (D–Oregon) called "the diet-business version of *Jaws*." There they were, three of the biggest weight-loss centers in the country, going at each other in court over a magazine article that ranked Nutri/System the best. Nutri/System has stopped touting the disputed rating, and the dust, at least in that skirmish, has settled.

But in this fiercely competitive industry, the grappling never really stops. A Jenny Craig ad displays a sleeked-down specimen happily showing off her trim new size 7 figure, down from size 18. Weight Watchers promises 15 pounds off in ten weeks with its new "Quick Control" program. Each year, more than eight million Americans sign up with structured weight-loss programs, paying hundreds and sometimes thousands of dollars, according to Marketdata Enterprises, a Valley Stream, New York, market research firm. Besides gunning for the postholiday resolution crowd, the big programs have been hammered by the recession—there were 9,444 commercial diet centers in 1989 and only 8,520 in 1991—and are aggressively fighting for market share, spicing up their pitches with incentives and sign-up bonuses.

What 7 Programs Offer

The philosophies of these commercial diet centers—and the fees they charge—span a wide range. A program that works for a friend may be all wrong for you. You want a plan you can afford, with an approach you can follow. These thumbnail descriptions of seven popular programs should help you make the best choice.

Diet Program	Diet Center	Jenny Craig
Number of centers	1,650	551
Phone number	(800) 333-2581	(800) 925-3669
Typical cost	$35–$50/week plus registration fee of under $100	$130 initially plus $3 per meal; $350 for life-time Success Plus program
Primarily group or individual?	Individual	Combination
Claim	2–3 pounds/week	1–2 pounds/week
Description	Reducing, conditioning and stabilizing diets. Nutrition, behavior-modification, weight and exercise counsel-ing. Your food or food provided by program. Body composition analysis at some centers.	Prepackaged foods plus vitamin supple-ment sold by the cen-ter, gradual weaning to regular food. Behavior modification, nutrition education, exercise plan, audiotapes for home use.
Schedule	6 days/week	Twice-weekly sessions
Staff	One week formal training, ongoing education	Counselors get 48 hours of training, con-tinuing education
Maintenance	One year of counseling	One year of monthly classes
Comments	New program is based on analysis of body composition and not on weight.	People who keep the weight off for a year and signed up for Success Plus get a 50 percent rebate.

Diet Program	Medifast	Nutri/System
Number of centers	10,000	Over 1,500
Phone number	(800) 535-3230	(800) 321-8446
Typical cost	$800–$2,000, depending on length of program	Sign-up fee of $108 (basic) to several hundred dollars (deluxe); $65/week for food
Primarily group or individual?	Individual	Combination
Claim	1–5 pounds/week	1½–2 pounds/week
Description	For those at least 20 pounds overweight. Total liquid diet or liquid diet plus some solid food, gradual weaning. Periodic medical testing. Behavior modification counseling. Exercise program.	Most food must be purchased at program center. Nutrition and behavior-modification classes. Exercise program. Customized programs for vegetarians, diabetics.
Schedule	Once a week	Once a week
Staff	Physician, other health professionals	College graduates with additional company training
Maintenance	Up to a year of classes	Regular counseling
Comments	Program varies from physician to physician. Possible side effects include lightheadedness, dizziness.	Up to 50 percent of sign-up fee for deluxe program rebated for keeping weight off for a year.

Optifast	Physicians Weight Loss Centers	Weight Watchers
350	Over 220	4,500
(800) 678-4327	(216) 666-7952	Check white pages
$85 weekly; total averages $3,000	$49–$500, plus $22 a week for supplements, depending on program	$18–$22 to register, plus $10–$12/week
Combination	Individual	Group
20 percent of body weight	½–3 pounds/week	1–2 pounds/week
For people 30 percent or more overweight. Liquid diet, solid food gradually reintroduced. Weekly group meetings, individual sessions with physician, behaviorist, dietitian.	Four meal plans geared to rate of loss, budget and supervision. Prepackaged food, not required. Nutritional supplements required. Nutrition, behavior and exercise counseling.	Support-group meetings feature behavior modification, nutrition education. Exercise program. Quick Control is a specified diet plan. Full Choice teaches you to put together your own diet.
Once a week	1–3 times weekly	Once a week
Physician, other health professionals	Doctor, other health professionals	Program graduates with extra training
6 months of biweekly classes	Weekly, 6–12 months	Weekly meetings
Possible side effects include dizziness, susceptibility to cold. Most centers are located in hospitals.	Everyone sees physician first. Biweekly visits for quickest weight loss.	Maintain loss for six weeks and you become a lifetime member, with no new registration fee.

Rating the Programs

Stripped down, the pitches are pretty much alike: a promise that you'll lose X pounds a week or month. The real difference is in how a program goes about it, and how well—but that's not easy to determine without signing up. You can get a quick sense of the quality by referring to the table on pages 241 to 243. The table gives capsule descriptions of the programs. As shown, some programs are oriented to groups, others to individuals. Some are run by health professionals, others by program "graduates." Clients may be limited to special foods or to a liquid diet purchased through the program or permitted store-bought food.

To succeed, you and the program have to match. You may value the camaraderie of a group, for example—or hate being one of a herd. Carol Delaney has lost 13 pounds in three months with Weight Watchers. The motivation she gets from the group sessions is "terrific," she says. Estelle Sciarrotta, on the other hand, hated the weekly weigh-in and the impersonality of the groups. "I tried Weight Watchers about 1,000 times," she says. "It just wasn't for me." Sciarrotta has lost 126 pounds on Optifast, a physician-directed program that provides a liquid diet and a more personal approach.

The ads don't help much. It's hard even to figure out how much the program will end up costing; the price of joining may be included, but you may have to buy special food at a cost that can far exceed the membership fee. And the ads are a major battleground for the companies. In 1990, Nutri/System advertised that it met American Heart Association guidelines, after asking for permission to make such a claim three years before and being turned down. The company halted its ad campaign at the request of the association's lawyers. Last year, Stanford University stopped Nutri/System from implying that the university endorsed the diet plan. And the company no longer boasts about last year's Number 1 ranking, which came from a *Healthline* magazine survey of 16 weight-loss programs. It turned out that the magazine had gotten a $25,000 "sponsorship fee" from Nutri/System after informing the company it had come out well in the survey. Jenny Craig and Weight Watchers sued the program for deceptive advertising. Nutri/System subsequently dropped the ad campaign.

Pseudoscience

Some ads make claims that sound scientific but are not. The Federal Trade Commission last fall forced NuDay Diet Program, which uses a protein powder and a fiber supplement, to stop claiming that the diet was capable of "altering metabolism" and "influencing mitochondrial activity" (the mitochondria are cells' source of energy) because the company couldn't demonstrate such a thing. (NuDay called it a disagreement over the "strength of the research.") More recently, the Federal Trade Commission has forced Ultrafast, Medifast and Optifast, which use doctor-supervised liquid diets, to tone down their ad claims and to back up future promises with hard data.

Overblown claims notwithstanding, all of the diet programs on the market really do work—at least for some people some of the time—if "work" is defined as losing weight. But a moment of triumph on the scales should not be the standard. "Anyone can lose weight," says David Garner, a Michigan State University psychologist and obesity specialist, "just like anyone can hold their breath." Keeping it off is something else. Nutritionists joke that owning a weight-loss franchise is great because of all the repeat business. But sooner or later, yo-yoing can discourage even the most stalwart dieters.

It could also kill them. A long-term survey of residents of Framingham, Massachusetts, reported in the *New England Journal of Medicine,* showed that people whose weight rose and fell repeatedly over a 32-year period had a

30 to 90 percent higher incidence of heart disease and early death than people whose weight remained stable. The excess is about the same as if the yo-yoers were simply obese. No one yet knows what could cause such an effect, but diet experts worry. "I'm afraid we're doing a lot of these people real harm," says Thomas Flynn, a doctor who says he quit as head of an Optifast program because so many clients kept cycling in and out of the program, regaining their lost weight and then losing it again.

It has made the whole question of going on a diet worth reconsidering. You may not need to lose weight anyway. "The vast majority of people who come to weight-loss programs don't have medical problems," says Lawrence Cheskin, director of Johns Hopkins Weight Management Center in Baltimore. That's why many insurance programs won't cover the cost of a diet program unless it was prescribed by a doctor, and some won't pay even then. For those whose diabetes, heart disease, high blood pressure, arthritis or other conditions are worsened by obesity, dropping just ten pounds may be enough to bring down blood pressure or eliminate the need for diabetes medication. Wayne Callaway, a physician who treats obese people, suggests using the ratio of your waist to your hips, not just your weight, as a rough indicator of the need to diet. The ratio for women should be about 0.75—for example, a waist measuring 30 inches and hips measuring 40—and for men the ratio should be 0.80 to 0.90. A higher number may be setting you up for high blood pressure, diabetes or atherosclerosis.

It doesn't take a costly program to lose weight and keep it off. Simply cutting down on fatty foods and upping your exercise—walking a little farther or faster than you do now—may be enough. Give it time; the U.S. Department of Agriculture suggests losing no more than a pound a week. Callaway warns that rapid weight loss can lead to gallstones or an obsession with thinness, resulting in anorexia or bulimia.

A Matter of Choices

For people who want guidance, weight-loss clinics at local hospitals or universities offer structured alternatives to commercial programs. "There's no one program that's best for everybody," says Johanna Dwyer, director of the Frances Stern Nutrition Center, a clinic and research division of New England Medical Center in Boston. "There's probably one best program for each individual, and it's no doubt not as good as we wish it would be."

It would be easier to choose a program if there were published studies that compared the relative benefits of different approaches, but such research doesn't exist. None of the big national programs can say how much weight, on average, their clients actually lose or whether it will stay lost. Based on studies of university programs, academics estimate that 10 percent of the participants on a very low-calorie liquid diet will have kept the weight off a year or two after completing the diet. This compares with a grim 5 percent for other methods.

Unlike medicines, diet programs like Jenny Craig and Weight Watchers don't fall under the scrutiny of the Food and Drug Administration, which considers them essentially menu plans. That means they don't have to demonstrate safety or effectiveness. They also go unscrutinized by national licensing or credentialing boards. Although you are on your own, you can subject a diet program to the following checklist, devised by three nutritionists at Baylor College of Medicine in Houston. Any good program should register six checks.

• An initial health screening, plus continuing supervision when there is heart disease or other medical risk
• An individual treatment plan with nutritional, exercise, educational and psychological components
• Full disclosure of the treatment plan and the step-by-step weight loss that is anticipated

- An ultimate weight goal based not on weight tables alone but also on personal and family history
- Psychological support along the way
- Emphasis on maintenance

Inconvenience can turn dieting from a bore to a chore. Daily attendance, a requirement of the Diet Center, might be difficult for parents with young children or for people who live 30 miles from the nearest center. But a nearby Diet Center might be just the thing for people who need frequent boosters to stick with it. Some people find that going through daily calculations of permissible meals on Weight Watchers' Full Choice plan provides both the constant reinforcement they need and a good way to learn about nutrition. Others find it odious—hence Weight Watchers' "Quick Control" alternative, which dictates specific meal plans and eliminates figuring. The required meals sold by Nutri/System and Jenny Craig may be a godsend for those who hate cooking, but anyone who regularly conducts business over lunch or dinner could soon fall off the diets. Nutri/System and Jenny Craig offer rebates on some registration fees if you keep the weight off for a year. That may be an inducement to some—and too much pressure for others.

Lowered Expectations

Surprisingly, dieters don't seem to care much about palatability. In a straw poll of a couple of dozen people who have gone through various programs, the only taste complaint concerned one cereal in the Jenny Craig program. Either the food is surprisingly good or dieters are resigned to expect less than haute cuisine.

Permanent success demands that you rewire your brain in significant ways. Judith Stern of the University of California at Davis compared women who maintained their weight loss for two years or more with women who yo-yoed. She found that the first groups of women had changed their attitudes about food, consistently selecting low-fat products; adopted a regular exercise program; and attacked problems rather than avoiding them even before setting out to lose weight.

These qualities can carry you through a slim life. "An obese person who loses weight is in remission, not cured," says Stern. For people who let their newly slim selves zombie out on late-night television with the chips and dip within arm's reach, that's food for thought.

Sweet Nothings Whispered in Your Ear—For about $10

"Diets do not work without personal commitment. Repeated playing of this tape could strengthen your desire, determination and willpower to effect a spectacular change now." So reads the label on an audiotape purported to "relax your conscious mind and cross the barrier to your subconscious"—that is, to get you to do what you've been unable to talk yourself into doing.

It's just one example of what are known as subliminal tapes, soundtracks of soothing music or nature sounds onto which manufacturers claim to put "hidden" messages—phrases and words recorded in such a way that they can't be picked up consciously ("stick to your diet," "eat less") but which your subconscious supposedly perceives and uses to bring about behavioral change. Americans spend more than $50 million annually on subliminal tapes and materials, often available in bookstores, health food shops and pharmacies for $10 or so and promoted for everything from losing weight to ending a cycle of procrastination to attracting a mate.

The notion that subliminal messages may influence behavior first became popular in the late 1950s when an advertising expert named James Vicary claimed to show the words "eat popcorn" and "drink Coke" for a third of a millisecond during the showing of the movie *Picnic*. The result, Mr. Vicary explained at the time, was that consumers purchased almost 60 percent more popcorn and nearly 20 percent more Coke.

Since then, he is reported to have admitted that his study was a hoax meant only to boost his faltering marketing business. But that hasn't stopped the ever-growing popularity of subliminal tapes. Nor have the findings of researchers who put subliminal tapes to the scientific test— and came up with no evidence that they are effective.

In one of the latest studies, more than 200 men and women listened for a month to tapes claimed either to build self-esteem or improve memory, the labels of which scientists varied so that some participants who thought they were hearing a self-esteem tape were actually listening to a memory tape and vice versa. The results? Not only were both types of tapes found to be ineffective, but some people who thought they had been listening to a memory tape and actually had been hearing a self-esteem tape were mistakenly convinced that their memory had improved. The same was true for several participants who believed they had been listening to a self-esteem tape but were in reality exposed to the sound of a so-called memory tape; they felt, incorrectly, that what they had been hearing bolstered their self-esteem.

"What you expect is what you believe, but it's not necessarily what you get," says one of the researchers involved, psychologist Anthony Pratkanis, Ph.D., of the University of California at Santa Cruz. His statement is supported by the findings of nearly a dozen other studies.

Research at the University of Northern Colorado, for instance, showed that people who listened to subliminal tapes designed to promote weight loss did not shed any more pounds over the course of eight weeks than people who did not hear the tapes. Adding to the evidence that subliminal self-help soundtracks are little more than a lucrative scam is a scientific analysis of tapes manufactured by four different companies. The researchers who investigated them found "no evidence whatsoever" that subliminal messages were ever recorded within the soundtracks. The message behind that message: The only thing tapes labeled subliminal appear to be truly capable of accomplishing is the parting of you and your money.

Reprinted with permission from *Tufts University Diet & Nutrition Letter*, 53 Park Place, 8th floor, New York, NY 10007.

Smoking Doesn't Solve Weight Problems: New Study Explodes Weight-Gain Myth

The most destructive weight-loss program ever devised has just gone up in a puff of smoke, thanks to results of a major new study.

You might call it the "lung-cancer diet"—when people cling to their cigarettes because they fear a large weight gain if they quit. New, definitive research, however, has shown that on average this weight gain is four pounds—a cinch to lose with a little exercise.

How little? Instead of walking a mile for a Camel, simply walk a mile—each day. A brisk 15-minute walk daily is all it takes to scale back that weight gain. And there are other benefits for ex-smokers in a stroll.

"It also improves your cholesterol profile and relieves the stress of nicotine withdrawal," says Ronald M. Davis,

M.D., director of the Office on Smoking and Health at the U.S. Centers for Disease Control, Rockville, Maryland. "Even if you do gain a few extra pounds, though, the effect on your health is nothing compared to the disastrous effects of smoking."

Earlier studies have suggested a much larger weight gain occurs after quitting. This latest study, though, reviewed all previous research that had been done—scanning the weight gains of over 20,000 quitters—to come up with this easily beatable four pounds.

FDA Bans Diet Pill Ingredients After Nearly 20 Years
By Frances M. Berg

Ever wonder about the safety of diet pills? Well, after more than 17 years' warning, the Food and Drug Administration (FDA) has announced a final date for banning 111 diet-pill ingredients not generally recognized as safe and effective for over-the-counter (OTC) sales.

The ban includes arginine, kelp, lysine and phenylalanine, often listed as ingredients in questionable diet products. Also banned is guar gum, which the FDA calls a safety hazard. After receiving reports of esophageal obstruction, the agency in July 1990 halted sales of Cal-Ban 3000, and has since taken action against other diet products containing guar gum.

Objections to the Ban

Companies promoting the banned ingredients filed five objections to the FDA action. They contend that regulating OTC weight control drug products is unconstitutional; that the FDA has no authority to regulate the purchase, sale, manufacture or labeling; and that consumers have the right of freedom of choice and a "health care" right to purchase any of these products.

In reply, FDA said: "Congress has concluded that the absolute freedom to choose an ineffective drug is properly surrendered in exchange for the freedom from the danger to each person's health and well-being from the sale and use of worthless drugs. . . . The surrender [of freedom of choice] is a rational decision which has resulted in achievement of greater freedom from dangers to health and welfare."

Monograph Possible

Since this is not the long-awaited monograph called for by frustrated FDA agents and the health community, the ban allows the possibility of other ingredients to be used, say officials. A monograph states which ingredients are allowable and bans *all* others.

The delay of a monograph on such an abused category of drugs is shocking, says Representative Ron Wyden (D–Oregon). "But given the chaotic state of research on obesity and weight control, this lapse was predictable."

FDA regional director Don Aird, of Minneapolis, is disappointed: "The most straightforward way to handle this would be to say, 'There are only two ingredients which are acceptable—anything else is not.' That's what a monograph is all about."

However, the FDA says this is a step toward a monograph.

With a new chief at the helm of the FDA there have been encouraging signs of the agency becoming more active in fighting fraud. David A. Kessler, M.D., who recently took over as commissioner, says, "People are being ripped off. We can't have an FDA inspector on every corner, but as an agency we'll do our part."

Dr. Kessler says he plans to crack down on purveyors of quack remedies.

PPA: Safe and Effective?

The ban does not include two other weight-control ingredients, phenylpropanolamine (PPA) and benzocaine, which were listed as safe and effective by the FDA in 1982. These are listed as ingredients in most weight-control pills found on grocery and drug-store shelves. For example, of 27 products listed in an "appetite suppressant product table" in the latest edition of the *Handbook of Nonprescription Drugs,* all contain either PPA or benzocaine. The FDA had reopened its investigation of PPA and benzocaine as nonprescription drugs for weight control. The agency is still accepting comments and reviewing information in regard to the safety, effectiveness and abuse of these two drugs.

Reprinted with permission from *Obesity and Health*, January/February 1992, pp. 10–11. Published by Healthy Living Institute.

Liquid Diets Suffer Another Blow to Their Image

Rarely has an individual so influenced the fortunes of an entire industry as Oprah Winfrey has weight-loss programs. Her gain was their loss.

But Oprah's announcement last year that she was happy heavier after gaining back most of the weight she lost on a liquid diet was just one in a series of jolts creating an image problem for very low-calorie diets—and the doctors who offer and monitor them.

The latest blow came when the Federal Trade Commission (FTC) charged three medically supervised liquid diet programs with misleading advertising.

The FTC actions follow congressional investigations into the diet industry, which also brought bad publicity.

"It's had an impact," said James Merker, executive director of Englewood, Colorado–based American Society of Bariatric Physicians (doctors who specialize in the study of obesity—its causes, treatment and prevention). The group, established 41 years ago, has seen membership fall to about 750 after reaching a peak of about 1,000 shortly after Oprah lost 67 pounds in late 1988.

Many of the physicians who have left the society were those who added liquid diets as an adjunct to their regular practice, Marker said. The society has always recommended tailoring diet programs to individual need using a variety of approaches.

Industry watchers confirm that sales of medically supervised diet programs have leveled off since early 1990 and that an industry shakeout is under way. They generally attribute sluggish sales to the recession and adverse publicity.

The FTC estimates that the programs still bring in about $600 million each year, a figure disputed by some firms that peg it lower, all part of a diet plan industry estimated at more than $2 billion.

About two thirds of the annual sales of medically supervised plans are estimated to go to the three programs named in the FTC agreements. Each markets very low-calorie liquid diets and other products through medical practices and hospitals. They are Optifast, marketed by Minneapolis-based Sandoz Nutrition Corp; Medifast, marketed by the Ownings Mills, Maryland–based Jason Pharmaceuticals and its subsidiary, Nutrition Institute of Maryland; and Ultrafast, marketed by Newington, Virginia–based National Center for Nutrition.

The proposed agreements will settle charges that the three companies "made deceptive and unsubstantiated claims regarding the safety and long-term efficacy of their programs."

The FTC will require the programs to disclose that the need for physician monitoring is to reduce risks associated with rapid weight loss. Also, when making claims about long-term weight loss, the programs must disclose sampling statistics for studies.

Bonnie Janesen, an FTC spokeswoman, acknowledged that at least a dozen other diet companies were under investigation, including commercial weight-loss centers and makers of over-the-counter products.

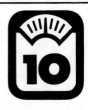

CHAPTER

10

THE FAT-FIGHTER'S MENUMATE: ALL YOUR FRIENDS AND ENEMIES EXPOSED

All You *Can* Eat

By now you know that the success of your weight-loss program depends largely on cutting dietary fat. You also know, from the Fat Goals table on page 21, how many grams of fat you can eat in order to achieve and *maintain* your ideal weight. This chapter will help you stick to your fat budget. How do you start? By doing these few simple things.

Read the "Fat Tag"

When you pick a food item off the shelf at the grocery store, make a habit of looking at the "fat tag," or nutrition label. If it doesn't meet your budgetary approval for fat content, put it back on the shelf, the same way you would if the price tag was too high.

Keep a Record

Each day, make a list of every food you eat and its fat content. As you choose your meals and snacks, keep a watchful eye on your fat tally for the day, and try not to exceed your goal. Pretty soon you will memorize how much fat your favorite foods contain.

Check the Table

To help you design your menu for the day, we've compiled the Fat-Fighter's MenuMate, beginning on page 260, which lists hundreds of everyday foods according to how much fat they contain in a serving.

When you choose your food according to how much fat you can "afford," you also find out how many extras you can eat. Have 10 grams of fat to spend at the end of the day? Pick out two 5s or a bit of chocolate for 9. Want to round out your breakfast with less than a gram of extra fat? Have half a cantaloupe, a peach or some grapes.

You'll be encouraged to see that the first category on the chart, "Foods with Less Than 1 gram of Fat," is the biggest. You may have learned from the Fat Goals table that you can eat 50 grams of fat a day, and at first that may not sound like much. But then browse this chart and look at all the great foods you *can* eat! There are lots of different foods that cost only 1 gram or less of your fat budget.

You'll also find a few surprises here. Some very popular snack foods like nuts and seeds, for example, are devastatingly high on the chart. A sweet, refreshing mango, on the other hand, will delight your mouth, satisfy your craving for a snack and fit perfectly into your fat budget.

So have fun browsing through this chart. Pick your snacks carefully and intelligently: Don't eat too many of those 0-grams-of-fat jelly beans!

THE FAT-FIGHTER'S MENUMATE

Food	Portion	Fat (g)

Foods with Less Than 1 Gram of Fat ◆

Food	Portion	Fat (g)
Arby's side salad	5.4 oz.	0
Burger King side salad	4.8 oz.	0
Chili sauce	1 Tbsp.	0
Diet nondairy creamer	1 packet	0
Egg substitute	¼ cup	0
Egg white	1	0
Gumdrops	1 oz.	0
Horseradish, prepared	1 Tbsp.	0
Jelly beans	1	0
Marshmallows	1 oz.	0
Popcorn, homemade, plain	1 cup	0
Relish	1 oz.	0
Soy sauce	1 Tbsp.	0
Teriyaki sauce	1 Tbsp.	0
White rice	½ cup	0
White rice, basmati	½ cup	0
Wild rice	⅓ cup	0
Angel food cake, from mix	2 oz.	0.1
Apricot, raw	1 (1.25 oz.)	0.1
Brown rice, basmati	½ cup	0.1
Carrot, raw	1 (2.5 oz.)	0.1
Celery	1 stalk	0.1
Chard, boiled	1 cup	0.1
Cornflakes cereal	1 cup	0.1
Cranapple juice	1 cup	0.1
Cranberry juice	1 cup	0.1
Cranberry sauce	¼ cup	0.1
Dill pickle	1	0.1
Evaporated skim milk	1 Tbsp.	0.1
Fruit cocktail	¼ cup	0.1
Ketchup	1 Tbsp.	0.1
Lettuce, romaine	1 cup	0.1
Peach	1	0.1
Pork gravy, from mix	1 Tbsp.	0.1
Prune juice	1 cup	0.1
Puffed rice cereal	1 cup	0.1

Food	Portion	Fat (g)
Radishes	6	0.1
Sweet pickle	1 small	0.1
Sweet potatoes, baked	4 oz.	0.1
Tamari sauce	1 Tbsp.	0.1
Tomato sauce, canned	¼ cup	0.1
Watercress	1 cup	0.1
Zucchini, boiled	1 cup	0.1
Alfalfa sprouts	1 cup	0.2
Animal crackers	1	0.2
Artichoke, boiled	4.2 oz.	0.2
Beets, canned	1 cup	0.2
Cabbage, red, raw	1 cup	0.2
Cauliflower, raw	1 cup	0.2
Figs, fresh	1 (0.75 oz.)	0.2
Grapefruit	1 (8 oz.)	0.2
Grape juice	1 cup	0.2
Lemon	1 (2 oz.)	0.2
Melon, casaba	1 cup	0.2
Orange, all varieties	1 (4.5 oz.)	0.2
Papaya	1 cup	0.2
Pineapple juice	1 cup	0.2
Potato, baked	1 (7 oz.)	0.2
Spinach, raw	1 cup	0.2
Apple juice	1 cup	0.3
Apples, dried	1 cup	0.3
Barbecue sauce	1 Tbsp.	0.3
Beef gravy, canned	1 Tbsp.	0.3
Broccoli, raw	1 cup	0.3
Cheese crackers	1	0.3
Chestnuts, roasted	1 oz.	0.3
Grapefruit juice	1 cup	0.3
Grapes	1 cup	0.3
Kiwifruit	1	0.3
Lettuce, iceberg	4.8 oz.	0.3
Mushrooms, raw	1 cup	0.3

(continued)

THE FAT-FIGHTER'S MENUMATE

Food	Portion	Fat (g)

Foods with Less Than 1 Gram of Fat (cont.)   ◆

Oyster crackers	5	0.3
Pepper, sweet	1 (2.6 oz.)	0.3
Rice cake	1	0.3
Sauerkraut, canned	1 cup	0.3
Squash, acorn, baked	1 cup	0.3
Sweet-and-sour dressing	1 Tbsp.	0.3
Syrup, chocolate flavor	1 oz.	0.3
Turkey gravy, canned	1 Tbsp.	0.3
Yellow mustard	1 Tbsp.	0.3
Broccoli, boiled	1 cup	0.4
Cabbage, boiled	1 cup	0.4
Cantaloupe	1 cup	0.4
Green or wax beans, boiled	1 cup	0.4
Mushroom gravy	1 Tbsp.	0.4
Onions, chopped	1 cup	0.4
Peas, boiled	1 cup	0.4
Plum, Japanese	1	0.4
Rye crackers	1	0.4
Skim milk	1 cup	0.4
Tuna, canned in water	3 oz.	0.4
Vegetable stock (soup), homemade	1 cup	0.4
Wheat crackers	1	0.4
Yogurt, nonfat	1 cup	0.4
Apple	5 oz.	0.5
Beef stock, canned	1 cup	0.5
Cottage cheese, low-fat (1%)	¼ cup	0.5
Garbanzo beans, canned	1 oz.	0.5
Graham crackers, plain	1	0.5
Grits (cereal)	1 cup	0.5
Lima beans, boiled	1 cup	0.5
Orange juice	1 cup	0.5
Asparagus, boiled	1 cup	0.6
Banana	1 (4 oz.)	0.6
Blackberries	1 cup	0.6
Blueberries	1 cup	0.6

Food	Portion	Fat (g)
Cream of Wheat hot cereal	1 cup	0.6
Mango	1 (7 oz.)	0.6
Nectarine	1 (5 oz.)	0.6
Pita pocket bread	1 (1.3 oz.)	0.6
Shredded wheat cereal	1 cup	0.6
Strawberries	1 cup	0.6
Tomatoes, canned	1 cup	0.6
Turkey, breast, roasted w/out skin	3 oz.	0.6
Vanilla wafer (cookie)	1 small	0.6
Yogurt cheese	1 oz.	0.6
Cherries, sour	1 cup	0.7
Oat flakes cereal	1 cup	0.7
Pear, Bartlett	1 (6 oz.)	0.7
Pineapple, diced	1 cup	0.7
Potato chip	1	0.7
Raisins	1 cup	0.7
Raspberries	1 cup	0.7
Shredded wheat cereal w/raisins	1 cup	0.7
Stroganoff sauce, mix	1 Tbsp.	0.7
Watermelon	1 cup	0.7
Wheat bran flakes cereal	1 cup	0.7
Brussels sprouts, boiled	1 cup	0.8
English muffin	1	0.8
Haddock, baked	3 oz.	0.8
Prunes	1 cup	0.8
Surimi (imitation crab)	3 oz.	0.8
Wheat bran flakes cereal w/raisins	1 cup	0.8
Wheat germ, toasted	1 Tbsp.	0.8
Brown rice	½ cup	0.9
Chicken gravy, canned	1 Tbsp.	0.9
Cracked wheat bread	1 slice (1 oz.)	0.9
Curry sauce, mix	1 Tbsp.	0.9
French, low-cal dressing	1Tbsp.	0.9
Lobster, steamed	3 oz.	0.9
Shrimp, steamed	3 oz.	0.9
White and mixed grain bread	1 slice (1 oz.)	0.9

(continued)

THE FAT-FIGHTER'S MENUMATE

Food	Portion	Fat (g)

Foods with 1 or More Grams of Fat ◆

Food	Portion	Fat (g)
Blue cheese, low-cal. dressing	1 Tbsp.	1.0
Bread, "lite" or diet	1 slice (1 oz.)	1.0
Brown mustard	1 Tbsp.	1.0
Corn, fresh, boiled	1 ear (2.7 oz.)	1.0
English muffin, oat bran	1	1.0
Fig bar (cookie)	1 average	1.0
Fudge cookie	1 small	1.0
Nondairy creamers, regular	1 Tbsp.	1.0
Oat bran bread	1 slice (1 oz.)	1.0
Pearl barley, dry	½ cup	1.0
Pretzel	1	1.0
Spaghetti or macaroni	1 cup	1.0
Split peas, dried, cooked	1 cup	1.0
Cheese sauce, mix, w/milk	1 Tbsp.	1.1
Oat cereal, "o-shaped"	1 cup	1.1
Spinach, canned	1 cup	1.1
Evaporated milk	1 Tbsp.	1.2
Nondairy whipped topping, frozen	1 Tbsp.	1.2
Scallops, steamed	3 oz.	1.2
Squid, raw	3 oz.	1.2
Bulgur, dry	½ cup	1.3
Corn bran cereal	1 cup	1.3
Crab, steamed	3 oz.	1.3
Hummus	1 Tbsp.	1.3
Saltines	5	1.3
Wheat bread	1 slice (1 oz.)	1.3
Bagel, egg or plain	1 (2 oz.)	1.4
Chicken stock, canned	1 cup	1.4
Ham, turkey	1 oz.	1.4
Taco sauce, canned	¼ cup	1.4
Bluefish, baked w/butter	3 oz.	1.5
Cherries, sweet	1 cup	1.5

Food	Portion	Fat (g)
Italian, low-cal dressing	1 Tbsp.	1.5
Tortilla, corn or flour	1	1.5
Asparagus, canned	1 cup	1.6
Corn, canned	1 cup	1.6
Gingersnap cookie, homemade	1 small	1.6
Tuna, canned, diet	3 oz.	1.6
Chicken liver pâté	1 Tbsp.	1.7
Clams, steamed	3 oz.	1.7
Flounder, baked	3 oz.	1.7
Half-and-half cream	1 Tbsp.	1.7
Onion soup, canned	1 cup	1.7
Red snapper, baked	3 oz.	1.7
Cheerios cereal	1¼ cups	1.8
Margarine, diet corn	1 tsp.	1.9
Parmesan cheese, grated	1 Tbsp.	1.9
Sour cream sauce, mix	1 Tbsp.	1.9
Tomato soup, canned w/water	1 cup	1.9
Vegetable beef soup, canned	1 cup	1.9
Vegetable soup, canned	1 cup	1.9
White sauce	1 Tbsp.	1.9

Foods with 2 or More Grams of Fat ◆

Food	Portion	Fat (g)
American cheese, singles	1 oz.	2.0
Brown 'n' serve roll	1 (1 oz.)	2.0
Canadian bacon, grilled	1 slice	2.0
Cream of mushroom soup, diet	10.5 oz.	2.0
Egg noodles	1 cup	2.0
Hard roll	1 (1.75 oz.)	2.0
Popcorn w/oil and salt	1 cup	2.0
Swiss cheese, light	1 oz.	2.0
Wendy's baked potato	8.8 oz.	2.0
Yogurt, frozen, fruit flavor	1 cup	2.0

(continued)

THE FAT-FIGHTER'S MENUMATE

Food	Portion	Fat (g)
Foods with 2 or More Grams of Fat (cont.)		◆
Marinara sauce, canned	¼ cup	2.1
Pancake from mix	1	2.1
Pastrami, turkey	1 oz.	2.1
Turkey or chicken roll, light or dark	1 oz.	2.1
Buttermilk	1 cup	2.2
Cucumber salad	¾ cup	2.2
Gazpacho, canned	1 cup	2.2
Taco shell	1	2.2
Tomatoes, stewed, homemade	1 cup	2.2
Venison, roasted	3.5 oz.	2.2
Chocolate sauce, homemade	1 Tbsp.	2.3
Chocolate/vanilla sandwich cookie	1 small	2.3
Clam chowder, Manhattan	1 cup	2.3
Figs, dried	1 cup	2.3
Chocolate chip cookie, from mix	1 small	2.4
Oatmeal	1 cup	2.4
Cottage cheese	¼ cup	2.5
French toast, frozen	1 slice	2.5
Halibut, broiled	3 oz.	2.5
Minestrone soup	1 cup	2.5
Hot fudge sauce, homemade	1 Tbsp.	2.6
Milk, low-fat (1%)	1 cup	2.6
Peanut butter cookie, from mix	1 small	2.6
Sour cream, imitation	1 Tbsp.	2.6
Chicken noodle soup, homemade	1 cup	2.7
Chocolate chip cookie, homemade	1 small	2.7
Margarine, whipped	1 tsp.	2.7
Chipped beef, dried	2.5 oz.	2.8
Light cream	1 Tbsp.	2.9
Olives, green or black	5	2.9

Food	Portion	Fat (g)

Foods with 3 or More Grams of Fat ◆

Food	Portion	Fat (g)
Caramel candy, plain and chocolate	1 oz.	3.0
Chicken breast, roasted w/out skin	½	3.0
Croutons	0.5 oz.	3.0
Fudge candy	1 oz.	3.0
Ham, baked	1 oz.	3.0
Onion ring, fried	1	3.0
Sour cream, cultured	1 Tbsp.	3.0
Spaghetti sauce, canned	¼ cup	3.0
Stuffing, prepared mix	½ cup	3.0
Bacon, fried or broiled	1 slice	3.1
Beef noodle soup, canned	1 cup	3.1
Gelatin, fruit-flavored	1 cup	3.1
Sponge cake, homemade	2.3 oz.	3.1
Turkey, leg, roasted w/o skin	3 oz.	3.2
McDonald's side salad	4.1 oz.	3.3
Peanut butter cookie, homemade	1 average	3.3
Potato salad, German	¾ cup	3.3
McDonald's chunky chicken salad	8.9 oz.	3.4
Sweet, candied, potato	1 (3.7 oz.)	3.4
Pancake, frozen	1	3.5
Yogurt, low-fat	1 cup	3.5
Margarine, soft, corn or safflower	1 tsp.	3.8
Margarine, stick, regular or corn	1 tsp.	3.8
Sherbet, orange	1 cup	3.8
Bagel w/lox and onion	1 (2 oz.)	3.9

Foods with 4 or More Grams of Fat ◆

Food	Portion	Fat (g)
Blueberry muffin	1 (2⅝″)	4.0
Burger King chunky chicken salad	9.2 oz.	4.0

(continued)

THE FAT-FIGHTER'S MENUMATE

Food	Portion	Fat (g)

Foods with 4 or More Grams of Fat (cont.) ◆

Food	Portion	Fat (g)
Corn muffin	1 (2⅝")	4.0
Gingerbread, mix	2.2 oz.	4.0
Hoagie roll	1 (4.75 oz.)	4.0
Mayonnaise, low-cal.	1 Tbsp.	4.0
Vienna sausage, canned, pork/beef	1 link	4.0
Yogurt drink	1 cup	4.0
Ham, extra lean	3 oz.	4.1
Pork tenderloin, roasted	3 oz.	4.1
Sardines, in oil	1.3 oz.	4.1
Biscuit	1 (2")	4.2
Oysters, on the half shell	3 oz.	4.2
Béarnaise or hollandaise sauce, mix	1 Tbsp.	4.3
Butterscotch sauce, homemade	1 Tbsp.	4.3
Vegetable soup w/barley	1 cup	4.4
Crab cake	1 (2 oz.)	4.5
Macaroon (cookie)	1 average	4.5
McDonald's cone, soft serve	3 oz.	4.5
Mozzarella cheese, part-skim	1 oz.	4.5
Chicken liver, simmered	3 oz.	4.6
McDonald's English muffin w/butter	1	4.6
Sardines, in tomato sauce	1.3 oz.	4.6
Soft ice milk	1 cup	4.6
Apple turnover	1 oz.	4.7
Olive loaf	1 oz.	4.7
Waffle, frozen	1	4.8
Blue cheese	1 oz.	4.9
Ricotta cheese, part-skim	¼ cup	4.9

Food	Portion	Fat (g)

Foods with 5 or More Grams of Fat ♦

Food	Portion	Fat (g)
Brownie with icing	1 oz.	5.0
Burger King garden salad	8 oz.	5.0
Cod, broiled w/butter	3.3 oz.	5.0
Haddock, breaded, fried	3 oz.	5.0
Lemon turnover	1 oz.	5.0
Long John Silver's ocean chef salad	8.4 oz.	5.0
Long John Silver's seafood salad	9.9 oz.	5.0
Wendy's garden salad	9.9 oz.	5.0
Bran muffin	1 (2⅝″)	5.1
Salmon, canned	3 oz.	5.1
Mayonnaise-style dressing	1 Tbsp.	5.2
London broil, top round	3 oz.	5.3
Corned beef	1 oz.	5.4
Mackerel, Atlantic, canned	3 oz.	5.4
Eye round roast	3 oz.	5.5
Heavy whipping cream	1 Tbsp.	5.5
Bologna, pork	1 oz.	5.6
Frog legs, fried	1 oz.	5.6
Raw or poached egg	1	5.6
Vanilla ice milk	1 cup	5.6
Brownie w/nuts, from mix	1 oz.	5.7
Ham and cheese loaf	1 oz.	5.7
Ranch-style dressing	1 Tbsp.	5.7
Salami, cooked beef	1 oz.	5.7
Toaster pastry	1	5.8
Bean soup w/bacon, canned	1 cup	5.9

(continued)

THE FAT-FIGHTER'S MENUMATE

Food	Portion	Fat (g)

Foods with 6 or More Grams of Fat ◆

Food	Portion	Fat (g)
Breakfast meat strips	3 strips	6.0
Cheesecake, low-cal.	4 oz.	6.0
Feta cheese	1 oz.	6.0
French or thousand island dressing	1 Tbsp.	6.0
Halibut, broiled w/butter	3 oz.	6.0
Leg of lamb, roasted, trimmed	3 oz.	6.0
Monterey Jack cheese, light	1 oz.	6.0
Pickle/pimiento loaf	1 oz.	6.0
Roy Rogers chicken leg	average	6.0
Swordfish, broiled w/butter	3.5 oz.	6.0
Tomato soup, canned w/milk	1 cup	6.0
Croissant, frozen	1	6.1
Mozzarella cheese, whole-milk	1 oz.	6.1
Pickled cabbage	½ cup	6.1
Corned beef hash	¼ cup	6.3
Squid, fried	3 oz.	6.4
Clam chowder, New England	1 cup	6.6
McDonald's garden salad	7.6 oz.	6.6
Neufchâtel cheese	1 oz.	6.6
Tortilla chips	1 oz.	6.6
French toast, homemade	1 slice	6.7
Liver, fried	3 oz.	6.8
Camembert cheese	1 oz.	6.9

Foods with 7 or More Grams of Fat ◆

Food	Portion	Fat (g)
Coffee cake, from mix	2.5 oz.	7.0
Pea soup, green, canned	1 cup	7.0
Pea soup, homemade	1 cup	7.0
Tuna, canned in oil	3 oz.	7.0

Food	Portion	Fat (g)
Gazpacho, homemade	1 cup	7.1
Scrambled egg w/milk and butter	1	7.1
Butter, whipped, tub	1 Tbsp.	7.3
Salmon, broiled w/butter	3.5 oz.	7.4
Yogurt, whole-milk	1 cup	7.4
French fried potatoes	3 oz.	7.5
Roy Rogers pancake platter	1	7.5
Blue cheese dressing	1 Tbsp.	7.6
Italian dressing	1 Tbsp.	7.6
Provolone cheese	1 oz.	7.6
Romano cheese	1 oz.	7.6
Russian dressing	1 Tbsp.	7.6
Chicken breast, roasted	½	7.7
Ham, roasted, w/bone	3 oz.	7.7
Gouda cheese	1 oz.	7.8
Swiss cheese	1 oz.	7.8
Brie cheese	1 oz.	7.9
Edam cheese	1 oz.	7.9
Oyster stew, canned, w/milk	1 cup	7.9
Tenderloin steak, broiled	3 oz.	7.9

Foods with 8 or More Grams of Fat ◆

Food	Portion	Fat (g)
Devil's-food cake, iced, mix	2.5 oz.	8.0
Instant breakfast drink	1 cup	8.0
Ricotta cheese, whole-milk	¼ cup	8.0
Shoulder of lamb, lean	3 oz.	8.0
Tapioca pudding, homemade	1 cup	8.0
Tartar sauce	1 Tbsp.	8.0
Vinegar and oil dressing	1 Tbsp.	8.0

(continued)

THE FAT-FIGHTER'S MENUMATE

Food	Portion	Fat (g)

Foods with 8 or More Grams of Fat (cont.) ◆

Waffle from mix	1	8.0
Liverwurst	1 oz.	8.1
Chitterlings (pork)	1 oz.	8.2
Rice pudding, w/raisins, homemade	1 cup	8.2
Whole milk	1 cup	8.2
Pastrami, beef	1 oz.	8.3
Brick cheese	1 oz.	8.4
Brownie w/nuts, homemade	1 oz.	8.5
Chocolate milk	1 cup	8.5
Muenster cheese	1 oz.	8.5
Pineapple upside-down cake, homemade	2.5 oz.	8.5
Arby's garden salad	8.8 oz.	8.6
Monterey Jack cheese	1 oz.	8.6
Rabbit, stewed	3 oz.	8.6
Ramen noodles	1 cup	8.6
Cauliflower soup, homemade	1 cup	8.7
Cheshire cheese	1 oz.	8.7
Roast beef, lean, trimmed	3 oz.	8.7
Roquefort cheese	1 oz.	8.7
Fontina cheese	1 oz.	8.8
American processed cheese	1 oz.	8.9
Mashed potatoes w/milk and butter	1 cup	8.9

Foods with 9 or More Grams of Fat ◆

Burger King chef's salad	9.8 oz.	9.0
Fudge brownie, microwave	1 oz.	9.0
Hash brown potatoes	½ cup	9.0

Food	Portion	Fat (g)
Milk chocolate bar	1 oz.	9.0
Taco Bell chili	9 oz.	9.0
Veal cutlet, broiled	3 oz.	9.0
Wendy's chef's salad	11.8 oz.	9.0
Colby cheese	1 oz.	9.1
Corn chips	1 oz.	9.1
Gruyère cheese	1 oz.	9.2
McDonald's hotcakes w/syrup	1 order	9.2
Cheddar cheese	1 oz.	9.4
McDonald's sundae, hot fudge	6 oz.	9.4
Duck, roasted w/out skin	3 oz.	9.5
McDonald's hamburger	1	9.5
Chicken leg, roasted w/out skin	1 (4 oz.)	9.6
Salami, hard	1 oz.	9.6
Celery soup, canned, w/milk	1 cup	9.7
Granola cereal, purchased	½ cup	9.8
Caramel sundae	6 oz.	9.9
Chicken capon, roasted	3 oz.	9.9
Clams, breaded, fried	3 oz.	9.9
Cream cheese	1 oz.	9.9
Roy Rogers roast beef sandwich	1	9.9
Scallops, breaded, fried	3 oz.	9.9

Foods with 10 or More Grams of Fat ◆

Food	Portion	Fat (g)
Burger King Chicken Tenders	6 pieces	10.0
Burger King vanilla shake	regular	10.0
McDonald's McLean Deluxe	1	10.0
Pot roast	3.5 oz.	10.0

(continued)

THE FAT-FIGHTER'S MENUMATE

Food	Portion	Fat (g)

Foods with 10 or More Grams of Fat (cont.) ♦

Food	Portion	Fat (g)
Vanilla pudding, homemade	1 cup	10.0
Sirloin steak, trimmed, broiled	3 oz.	10.1
McDonald's vanilla shake	regular	10.2
Semisweet chocolate bar	1 oz.	10.2
Taco Bell burrito, bean	1	10.2
Fish sticks, frozen	3 (1 oz.)	10.3
Homemade chicken stock	1 cup	10.3
Shrimp, breaded, fried	3 oz.	10.4
Oysters, fried	3 oz.	10.7
Chocolate bar w/peanuts	1 oz.	10.8
Lobster, broiled w/butter	1 tail (5 oz.)	10.8
Taco Bell taco	1	10.8
Hot fudge sundae	6 oz.	10.9

Foods with 11 or More Grams of Fat ♦

Food	Portion	Fat (g)
Arby's chef's salad	11.1 oz.	11.0
Chow mein noodles	1 cup	11.0
Mayonnaise	1 Tbsp.	11.0
Perch, breaded, fried	3 oz.	11.0
Coleslaw	½ cup	11.1
Taco Bell tostada	1	11.1
Doughnut, glazed	1	11.2
Lemon meringue pie, homemade	4 oz.	11.2
Trout, brook	3.5 oz.	11.2
Butter, regular, stick	1 Tbsp.	11.4

Food	Portion	Fat (g)
Cream of chicken soup, canned	1 cup	11.5
McDonald's french fries	regular	11.5
Sausage links, low-fat	2–3	11.5
Pastrami, turkey, sandwich on wheat	1	11.6
Pork loin, trimmed, roasted	3 oz.	11.6
Rib steak	3.5 oz.	11.6
Rib roast, trimmed	3 oz.	11.7
McDonald's Egg McMuffin	1	11.9
Rice, crispy cereal	1 cup	11.9

Foods with 12 or More Grams of Fat ◆

Food	Portion	Fat (g)
Banana cream pie, homemade	4.5 oz.	12.0
Burger King apple pie	1	12.0
Chocolate-covered peanuts	1 oz.	12.0
Chocolate pudding, homemade	1 cup	12.0
Peanuts, honey roasted	1 oz.	12.0
Roy Rogers breakfast crescent	1	12.0
Tofutti	1 cup	12.0
Salmon patty	3.5 oz.	12.4
Beef or pork frankfurter w/cheese	1	12.5
Waffle, homemade	1	12.6
Corned beef, canned	3 oz.	12.7
McDonald's biscuit w/spread	1	12.7
Lard	1 Tbsp.	12.8
Pork shoulder, lean, roasted	3 oz.	12.8
Vegetable shortening	1 Tbsp.	12.8
Ham, canned, roasted	3 oz.	12.9

(continued)

THE FAT-FIGHTER'S MENUMATE

Food	Portion	Fat (g)

Foods with 13 or More Grams of Fat ◆

Burger King french fries	regular	13.0
Pork chop, trimmed	3 oz.	13.0
Snickers chocolate bar	2 oz.	13.0
Mackerel, broiled w/butter	3 oz.	13.4
Olive oil	1 Tbsp.	13.5
Apple pie, homemade	5 oz.	13.6
Corn oil	1 Tbsp.	13.6
Cream of mushroom soup	1 cup	13.6
Danish pastry, plain	1	13.6
Eclair, custard-filled, iced	3.5 oz.	13.6
McDonald's chef's salad	10.1 oz.	13.6
Safflower oil	1 Tbsp.	13.6
Ground beef, 10% fat	3 oz.	13.9
Roy Rogers breakfast crescent w/bacon	1	13.9

Foods with 14 or More Grams of Fat ◆

Burger King bagel w/egg and cheese	1	14.0
Custard pie, homemade	4.5 oz.	14.0
Hardee's garden salad	8.6 oz.	14.0
McDonald's McLean Deluxe w/cheese	1	14.0
Veal rib, roasted	3 oz.	14.0
10% fat ice cream	1 cup	14.3
Turkey club sandwich on whole wheat	1	14.3
McDonald's apple pie	1	14.8

Foods with between 15 and 20 Grams of Fat ◆

Arby's roast-beef sandwich	1	15.0
Blueberry pie, homemade	5 oz.	15.0

Food	Portion	Fat (g)
Cherry pie, homemade	5 oz.	15.0
Custard, baked	1 cup	15.0
Hardee's chef's salad	10.5 oz.	15.0
Pumpkin pie, homemade	4.5 oz.	15.0
Spinach, creamed, frozen	4.5 oz.	15.0
Wendy's french fries	regular	15.0
Chocolate cream pie, homemade	3.5 oz.	15.1
Avocado, Florida	1 (6 oz.)	15.4
Chicken leg, roasted	1 (4 oz.)	15.4
Ground beef, 21% fat	3 oz.	15.7
Burger King onion rings	regular	16.0
Cheesecake	3 oz.	16.3
McDonald's Chicken McNuggets	4 oz.	16.3
Beef or pork frankfurter	1	16.6
Granola cereal, homemade	½ cup	16.6
Crab, imperial	1 cup	16.7
Pound cake, homemade	2 oz.	17.2
Taco Bell burrito, beef	1	17.3
Ground beef, 30% fat, baked or broiled	3 oz.	17.8
Roy Rogers chicken breast	average	18.0
Wendy's sausage patty w/out gravy	1 patty	18.0
Chicken breast, batter-fried	½	18.5
Roast beef sandwich on rye	1	18.8

(continued)

THE FAT-FIGHTER'S MENUMATE

Food	Portion	Fat (g)

Foods with between 15 and 20 Grams of Fat (cont.)

Food	Portion	Fat (g)
Knockwurst, pork/beef	1 (2.4 oz.)	18.9
Potato salad, w/mayonnaise	¾ cup	18.9
Burger King Croissan'wich	1	19.0
Wendy's breakfast sandwich	1	19.0
Wendy's chicken sandwich	1	19.0
Wendy's french toast	2 slices	19.0
Arthur Treacher's chicken sandwich	1	19.2
Ground beef, 30% fat, fried	3 oz.	19.2
Roy Rogers roast beef sandwich w/cheese	1	19.7
Arthur Treacher's fish	5.2 oz.	19.8

Foods with between 20 and 30 Grams of Fat ◆

Food	Portion	Fat (g)
Chef's salad, no dressing	average	20.1
McDonald's Quarter Pounder	1	20.7
Homemade beef stock	average	21.0
Wendy's chicken nuggets	6 pieces	21.0
Wendy's omelet w/cheese and ham	1	21.0
Bagel w/cream cheese	1 (2 oz.)	21.1
Greek salad, w/feta cheese	average	21.5
Arthur Treacher's chicken	4.8 oz.	21.6
Arby's Super	1	21.7
Italian, pork sausage	3 oz.	21.8
Bratwurst (sausage)	3 oz.	22.0
Soft ice cream	1 cup	22.5

Food	Portion	Fat (g)
Taco Bell taco bellgrande	1	23.0
Kielbasa (sausage)	3 oz.	23.1
Vanilla ice cream	1 cup	23.7
Arthur Treacher's fish sandwich	1	24.0
Burger King Croissan'wich w/bacon	1	24.0
Wendy's potato w/sour cream and chives	10.9 oz.	24.0
Duck, roasted	3 oz.	24.1
Coconut, dry, flaked	1 cup	24.4
Polish pork sausage	3 oz.	24.4
Wendy's potato w/broccoli and cheese	12.9 oz.	25.0
Macaroni salad	½ cup	25.1
Spareribs (pork), braised	3 oz.	25.7
McDonald's Fillet o' Fish	1	26.1
Tuna salad	⅓ cup	26.1
Lobster, Newburg	1 cup	26.5
Lobster, thermidor	5.5 oz.	26.6
Coconut, raw, shredded	1 cup	26.8
Burger King Whaler	1	27.0
Eggs, sausage, and hash browns, frozen	5.5 oz. pkg.	28.0
Taco Bell taco, light	1	28.8
Burger King french toast sticks	1 order	29.0

(continued)

279

THE FAT-FIGHTER'S MENUMATE

Food	Portion	Fat (g)

Foods with between 20 and 30 Grams of Fat (cont.)

McDonald's biscuit w/sausage	1	29.1
McDonald's Quarter Pounder w/cheese	1	29.2

Foods with between 30 and 40 Grams of Fat ◆

Avocado, California	1 (6 oz.)	30.0
Chicken-fried steak	3.5 oz.	30.0
Arby's fish fillet	1	30.9
Burger King bacon double cheeseburger	1	31.0
Grilled cheese sandwich	1	31.0
Lamb chop, broiled	3 oz.	32.0
McDonald's Big Mac	1	32.4
Turkey club sandwich on white	1	33.5
Wendy's baked potato w/cheese	12.3 oz.	34.0
Roast beef w/mayonnaise, on rye	1	35.1
McDonald's biscuit w/egg	1	35.3
Arby's Bacon 'n Cheddar Deluxe	1	35.7
Mousse, chocolate, homemade	⅔ cup	35.7
Burger King bagel w/sausage	1	36.0
Burger King Great Danish	1	36.0
Burger King Whopper	1	36.0
Pastrami, beef, sandwich on rye	1	36.0
Arby's cashew chicken salad	13.4 oz.	37.0
Wendy's taco salad	28.3 oz.	37.0

Food	Portion	Fat (g)
Ham and cheese sandwich on rye	1	37.7
Chicken salad	⅔ cup	39.0
Wendy's Big Classic Double	1	39.0
Burger King chicken specialty	1	40.0

Foods with More Than 40 Grams of Fat ◆

Egg salad	½ cup	41.0
McDonald's McD.L.T.	1	42.1
Burger King Whopper w/cheese	1	43.0
Wendy's Bacon Swiss burger	1	44.0
Tuna/cheese melt (sandwich)	1	48.2
Wendy's sausage patty w/gravy	1 patty	54.0
Chef's salad	average	56.1
Reuben sandwich grilled, on rye	1	59.5
Taco Bell taco salad	20.5 oz.	61.0
Hero (sandwich)	1	62.2
Cashews, dry roasted	1 cup	63.5
Pistachio nuts, dry roasted	1 cup	67.6
Almonds, dry roasted, whole	1 cup	71.3
Sunflower seeds, dried	1 cup	71.4

(continued)

THE FAT-FIGHTER'S MENUMATE

Food	Portion	Fat (g)

Foods with More Than 40 Grams of Fat (cont.) ◆

Food	Portion	Fat (g)
Sesame seeds, dried	1 cup	71.5
Filberts (hazelnuts)	1 cup	72.0
Pecans	1 cup	73.1
Walnuts, English	1 cup	74.2
Peanuts, dry roasted w/out salt	1 cup	76.5
Sunflower seeds, oil-roasted	1 cup	77.6
Brazil nuts	1 cup	92.7
Macadamia nuts	1 cup	98.8

Sources: Food Values: Cholesterol and Fats by Leah Wallach; U.S. Department of Agriculture; National Research Council; manufacturers' data.

Index